Raising Jennica

Janet Johnson-Thonen

H. Habascrab Publishing
Oberlin, OH

Raising Jennica

ISBN 978-0-615-47835-7

Library of Congress Registration Number: TX 7-425-995

Dedication

To Jennica with love and hope. To my children Julie, Joshua, and Jonna for blessing my life. To John who traveled this journey with me. Much love to all of you. This is your story too.

Contents

Raising Jennica

Foreword

I would love to say that this is a "...they lived happily ever after..." story. It isn't. It is a story of a life apart. It is a story about the pain of discrimination sweetened by people who offered compassion and love. It is the story of my daughter Jennica's life and the family that surrounded her. I share it to give her a legacy. To give her a voice. I asked Jennica if she would like a book written about her and she said, "Yes. I would like a book that tells how difficult my disabilities have made my life." This is that book.

A Birthday

It was raining on the gray day Jennica was born. We drove through its sad song on the way to the hospital as the windshield wipers swished back and forth, back and forth. It didn't bother me. The radio in our Beetle was playing cheerful music and we were singing along, happy that this was the day our child would be born. I was tired of the stares from strangers who felt free to ask if I was pregnant with twins or bluntly told me I should be home in "my condition". The doctors told me the baby was at least nine pounds and I looked it. I was huge. So this was a happy day, but perhaps the rain was trying to tell me something.

I was being induced. I was overdue and the doctor felt I was ready. It was 1973 and on that gloomy February day I was delighted that my doctor had decided it was time. I trusted the doctor. I trusted the world of medicine. I was young, I was naive, and this gray day was the last for me to be either.

Nurses started the drugs which dripped from the IV hanging overhead. I was in a fresh hospital gown, tucked into the crisp sheets of a hospital bed and my eager husband, John, couldn't stop smiling. At first all seemed well. My labor started almost immediately and from the beginning the pains were strong. John was making silly jokes about us being a baby making machine. The nurses believed our child would arrive soon and so, in between pains, we laughed.

As the hours passed, it ceased being fun and the laughter stopped. The pains were unbearable and I was not progressing. The doctors sent me for X-rays to see if I could safely deliver this child. I knew then there was trouble and for the first time I began questioning the medical profession. I had been sent for X-rays the day before by the same doctors. For the same reason. I told them that and I was ignored.

A monitor was attached to record the baby's heart rate. With each contraction it dropped into the forties and then rebounded. Hours passed with no progress and with no relief from the intense pain. When the baby's heart rate dropped even lower, the doctor appeared and I was rushed into surgery for an emergency cesarean section. I was given general anesthesia and the doctor delivered Jennica.

She weighed eleven pounds two ounces and was twenty three inches long. She had long black hair and the sweetest little mouth possible. She also had an Apgar of 4, low muscle tone, and poor color. When tested again thirty minutes later, it remained the same.

John saw her briefly. He said her skin was bluish tinged. He also said she was beautiful. No one told him there was a problem and so he called family to tell them how big and beautiful his new daughter was. I had a tube down my throat, oxygen flowing into my nose, IVs dripping into my veins, and I was catheterized. Through this maize I vaguely heard that I had a daughter. I saw her later, for just a brief moment, and by then her color was rosy. I was stunned by her size and by how lovely she was. People were peeking into my room, smiling, laughing, and saying they wanted to see the woman who delivered the big, beautiful, baby.

I was happy that night. Drugged, but happy, and in a morphine mist I drifted away. Morning brought the removal of some tubes and rounds of doctors. I was still happy. I remember feeling that if I died right then and there, it would be fine. Hormones, or the morphine perhaps, but I was euphoric. It was a happiness that couldn't last. Nothing that perfect ever does.

The doctors began questioning me about my pregnancy. They ran tests for diabetes, for low calcium, for infections. They began expressing concerns. Not for me, but for the source of my happiness, Jennica. She was trembling they told me. Her limbs, her sweet rosebud mouth; they trembled. Her head size worried them. Her difficulty with nursing bothered them. My dreamlike happiness became a nightmare that I couldn't wake up from and no one would look me in the eye and tell me the truth.

I remember lying in bed the third morning, crying. Though no one would tell me anything, I knew there was a problem. I didn't know how severe, and I didn't know exactly what, but I knew everyone was concerned about my beautiful daughter. I heard the nurses whispering about it. I saw it in their eyes. I knew the doctors' questions were not idle curiosity. And so I cried, and into those tears walked a new doctor. A doctor that would become Jennica's pediatrician, her advocate, and defender. He looked straight at me and asked me what was wrong and why I was worried. I told him and he tried to explain what might be going on with her. He wasn't certain but he thought perhaps she had a condition called transient cerebral edema. It would explain the trembling and the poor muscle tone. He was cautiously optimistic but he was going to follow her closely. And then he told me that my daughter was lovely.

Though the doctor who delivered Jennie never again saw her or visited me, this new doctor taught me that there were indeed good people in medicine. That there were compassionate people in medicine. And on that I hung my hope.

Homecoming

After a week in the hospital, I convinced the doctors to discharge me. I had complications from the surgery but I felt I needed to be home, so with the assurance that I would have help, they let me go. Jennica was released at the same time and I was delighted we were returning to our apartment with our daughter. Jennie's room was a cheerful haven, just waiting for her. John and I had transformed it into a sunny jungle with trees, a smiling sun, and animals covering the walls. Bright yellow curtains hung over her windows and her white furniture was full of sweet baby clothes. With our fingers crossed, John tucked Jennica into her new car seat and off we went. We went with smiles on our faces and a beautiful baby girl in the backseat. Heading off to a life that we couldn't even imagine and certainly hadn't planned, but on that day we felt nothing but joy.

My family waited for us at our home. They had visited us at the hospital but they were anxious to hold and inspect their new granddaughter up close. My father held her and told me what good work I had done. My youngest brother, Tim, was delighted by his new niece and my mother was staying, helping to take care of her for a week. They all took turns holding her and admiring her dark beauty. My family is fair and this new member of the clan was rather exotic with her rosy skin and long dark hair. Jennie was also greeted by our dog and cat. Yuki, a small American Eskimo, sniffed Jennica's pretty head and fell in love. Nina, our lovely, gray, long haired cat, tiptoed around her and ran for cover when Jennie kicked her little feet. We laughed and smiled and felt complete.

My mother kept Jennica with her in the living room that week. Mom slept on the pullout couch and Jennie slept in her bassinet. That bassinet was special. White wicker with a dainty white and yellow liner, it also had a history. Twenty four years before Jennica slept in that bassinet, I had slept there. And then my brothers rested there. First Robert, then William, and finally, my youngest brother Timothy. Now, the family's first grandchild slept there, and sleep she did. We were all delighted that she was eating well and sleeping through the night. My mother enjoyed her time with her new granddaughter and I rested, as the doctors had ordered. I remained concerned but looking at my sweet daughter, I was hopeful.

Soon it was time for my mother to return home. She had a job she needed to return to and my father missed her. I was still weak but felt I could take care of Jennie with John's help at night after work. We settled into a routine. Because she wouldn't nurse, we bottle fed her. John would feed her before he left for work, burp her, and leave for the office with formula covering his shoulder. I sat and rocked her in the wooden rocking chair that we had painted a soft blue. I rocked and sang, happy with my baby in my arms. The fear I had felt in the hospital never really left, but I was hopeful that all would be well. When I looked into her face I could see nothing but her beauty.

I bundled Jennica up in warm clothes and blankets on a bright but chilly day in the middle of March. I wore the only shoes that fit. Though I had lost the weight of pregnancy, my legs and feet remained swollen. Too swollen to wear appropriate shoes. So, Jennica in her fuzzy blankets, and me in my sandals, headed off to see her pediatrician for her two week check up. John was at work and was not able to join us, so we traveled by cab. Her smiling doctor and his staff scolded me for dressing her too warmly and began unwrapping my darling girl. Then they weighed her, measured length and head size, asked developmental questions, and closely observed her. This was to become a routine for us. Frequent visits were scheduled and Jennica's progress was charted and discussed. Though we had no idea what the future held, we remained optimistic. All of us. The visits were important to me for support and for answers to my growing questions. This first visit ended on a positive note and I taxied home with a sprig of hope.

The early weeks with Jennica were sweet, even with a tinge of worry. She smiled and appeared happy and alert. She grew rapidly, not even falling on the normal growth charts for infants. She lost some of her early chubbiness and became long and thin. She ate well but it only seemed to help her grow long bones and long hair. John and I referred to her as our "home entertainment center" and each night we set up an elaborate bath for her, watching her relax and splash in the warm water. We smoothed her skin with lotions and dressed her in nightgowns. Her little feet peeked out and we never tired of admiring every inch of her.

I had fun dressing her up and showing her off to family when they visited or when we drove to my hometown. We did that often, staying with my parents for the night and sleeping in my childhood room. Mom had purchased a crib sized playpen that Jennica slept in, close to our bed. We split our time between our families and they all enjoyed holding Jennie and watching the changes in her from visit to visit. Her uncles and aunts adored her but they worried. We all worried.

As she grew it became more and more apparent that Jennie had low muscle tone. We waited for her neck to become strong enough to support her head, but it wobbled and bobbled. We tried to laugh and tell ourselves, all in good time, but we knew it wasn't okay. One sad day we took her for her first studio photos. We put her in a lacey, soft yellow dress and we thought she looked lovely. There was a baby girl the same age as our Jennie being photographed first. This infant held her head up and her body seemed so strong and firm as they posed her and snapped her picture. Then it was Jennica's turn. What had seemed so effortless for the previous baby was simply impossible for her. I remember feeling as if I couldn't breathe. I remember "knowing" Jennica was not okay. That this was not going to turn out just fine. I remember feeling the beginning of a sadness that would last a lifetime.

All parents watch their children grow. They do it with love and concern. We did the same but we did it more carefully. I noted and recorded each milestone, knowing that her doctor would ask, and chart. And just in case I was stretching the truth he would observe her for long periods of time in his office. Would she pass the keys from one hand to another? Would she startle at a clap she couldn't see? Would she reach for objects that interested her? Did she coo? Did she roll over? Did she hold up her head when placed on her stomach? It is a delight to see your children develop but when you have a child that is at risk it is also stressful, and sometimes heartbreaking. We held our breath. Our doctor did the same. And we all hoped and prayed.

There were good times when she was little. She would reach for and laugh at our dog. Her laugh was huge and low in pitch. We wondered if her voice would be low when she learned to speak. She loved her baths and kicked and smiled. She was fearless and loved each and every person that held her. She assumed that everyone adored her and she was right.

She learned to crawl before she turned one. She called us Mama and Dada. We were hopeful but we never relaxed. We bought her toys and she quickly learned how they worked, impressing us and all those around her. I remember thinking maybe this will just be a problem with her muscles. Just a little problem. A little delay. Jennica's doctor expressed the same hope. There was definitely a problem with her muscle tone. It was low and it made her movements look awkward. She began walking around furniture when she was a little over a year but she couldn't let go. She couldn't walk on her own. We took her to an orthopedic doctor who prescribed special shoes for her to give her support. They were bigger and heavier than normal baby shoes and sometimes I thought perhaps they were the problem instead of a solution.

The Christmas she was twenty two months she was still not walking. She was lovely then. Dark brown hair with rosy skin and big brown eyes. She had a smile on her face whenever you looked at her and she was a happy child. But she didn't walk. That Christmas we gave her a Raggedy Ann doll and a chime ball. It was musical and had little horses and figures inside of it. When it moved, it chimed out a tinkling melody. Jennie loved that ball and so we used it to encourage her to begin walking. We would throw it just beyond her and then stand her up. And she walked, smiling and laughing. She walked to get that beautiful, magical, toy. We held our breath. We grinned. We clapped. We hugged her and we shed happy tears for a milestone that had seemed so elusive. Jennica? She just smiled that huge smile and continued to walk. It was our very own Christmas miracle.

Miracles are in short supply and to expect many more would have been irrational. Instead we worked on helping Jennica grow and develop. We purchased educational toys that offered stimulation. We supported her through play and love. The doctor continued to closely monitor her development. Through it all the smile stayed on her pretty face and so she encouraged us as we encouraged her.

It was a nice time. We shared a duplex with another young family. The mother became my friend and Jennica's cheerleader. She showed Jennie both love and acceptance, and her children did the same. During the day while our husbands were building their careers, we were busy with our families. My friend would often scoop Jennie up and take her into her kitchen for a treat. She would peel grapes for her or give her cookies. She made popcorn and took the kernels apart for Jennie. These little acts of kindness helped both Jennie and myself. While she understood Jennica's problems, she also saw the delightful person she was. And she loved her. Alone in a new city with no family, I needed a support system and our neighbors supplied it. Her husband and John became friends and the duplex we shared became one big family. For almost two wonderful years our lives were intertwined and then we began considering another child.

Our New Home and Growing Family

We had always planned on a large family. We thought perhaps two biological and two adopted children. It seemed like a wonderful plan and as Jennica grew, the idea grew too. It had not been suggested that Jennie's problems were genetic, so we thought that all would be fine with the next pregnancy. First we needed more space and so we decided to buy a home. Having served in the military, John was eligible for a VA loan. That meant no down payment and low rate financing would be available. So with Jennica secure in the backpack we set out looking for our first home.

We wanted a nice yard, three bedrooms, and a safe neighborhood. It didn't take us long to find a cute brick ranch in a nice suburb. It was cozy but had plenty of room for Jennica and another child. The yard had lovely and varied plantings making it a lush garden retreat for all of us. Buying a home was easy but leaving our new friends was not. We knew they too would soon be looking for a house but it was difficult to be the first to depart. So with a combination of tears and excitement we moved on.

The house was made with a circular pattern and Jennica would run around the parameter time after time, never tiring of the fun. Sometimes Yuki ran with her, having a little fun too. John and I found our enjoyment came from decorating the house and we started with Jennie's room. Wallpaper was very popular then and so we covered her walls with pretty pink flowered paper. I made soft pink curtains to cover her windows and her new "big girl" bed stood proudly in the space. She loved her new room and when we set up all of her Fisher Price toys, she was overjoyed. For hours on end she would arrange the people, the houses, and villages. Little people would be put into vehicles and driven around her miniature neighborhood. Sometimes we played with her but she was also content to play alone. She had a wonderful imagination and watching her, we were hopeful.

Of course we didn't like everything we observed. Jennie still had the low muscle tone that had been present since birth and the doctors had finally decided she had a form of cerebral palsy. So we now had a label, but it just gave us something to write in the blanks when we filled out forms for her. It didn't change anything. It didn't give us a prognosis or a way to help her. It simply gave a name to a problem we knew existed.

Her speech was also slightly delayed. While she was able to say many words, they weren't strung together in sentences. Her voice was low and a little rough, no doubt a result of the muscle tone problems, making her sometimes difficult to understand. At around two years of age I requested she see a speech therapist and her pediatrician, always eager to help, gave us the name of a family friend, a young woman with a small daughter of her own. She came to our house twice a week and helped Jennie become more fluent. She did a marvelous job and Jennica was very fond of her. Before she started speech therapy Jennie had begun acting frustrated when we could not understand her. With just a few months of help she improved and once again became her cheerful self.

While most young children become ill with colds and ear infections, Jennica became ill more often and more seriously. I often made a bed on the floor of her room where I could be close to her and watch over her. One morning, after a long sleepless night with Jennie crying and coughing, she was so ill she could not even sit up. She simply lay on the floor - listless and quiet. It frightened me and I dressed her and drove her to the doctor. After tests were run they determined that she had pneumonia and that it was effecting her heart. They gave her medication and sent her home hoping to avoid hospitalizing her. The doctors must have chosen the right medicine because in a few hours she was feeling so much better that it shocked me. It also rather shocked me that her doctor called to check on her. While I trusted and respected her pediatrician, I still maintained a basic distrust of the medical profession, and to hear the concern in the doctor's voice, surprised and touched me.

John and I were still worried by the tests that had shown her heart was enlarged and we held our breath until she was well and they could check her again. Sometimes we talked about our worries. Sometimes I cried. Long nights lying in bed thinking about her health were much too frequent. I would tell God that I could handle her having disabilities but I couldn't handle losing her. So I prayed. Finally the day for her recheck arrived, and with it good news. Her heart looked normal. We could breathe. We could smile! We seldom heard good news about Jennie's health and we savored the moment.

It was a happy time for us. I was pregnant with our second child, which brought us both excitement and a little anxiety. We enjoyed our life with Jennica though it was not how we had pictured our life with children. This life had too many doctor appointments and too many worries about our child's future. But it was the life we had been given and we still found sweet moments in each day with nothing sweeter than the smiles our daughter showered over us. Now we kept our fingers crossed and we hoped for the best, carefully happy about the new baby that was coming.

One evening in February, two weeks before Jennie turned two, I miscarried. I was twelve weeks along. The physical pain I felt in the hospital was insignificant compared to the pain in my heart. It seemed a burden too big to bear. I had been calm and accepting of Jennica's problems but I wasn't sure I could face losing this child. Of course I had no choice. No choice at all. And so I returned home from the hospital with a new hurt that I hadn't seen coming. John was as sad as I was. He had wanted to fill our house with children and this dream was starting to seem impossible.

We did go on. We convinced ourselves that this wouldn't happen again. We concentrated on Jennica and making sure she was happy. At the end of February family and friends came to celebrate her birthday. It was a rare day, unseasonably warm, and we went outside without coats to pose for a family picture. Later I would look at the photo and feel as if I could almost see my lost child. I wore a smile but my eyes were as empty as my arms.

Losing the baby moved us forward in our plans for adoption. We had always planned to adopt. The first year of our marriage we boldly decided to have two biological children and to adopt two more. I say boldly because in the flush of youth and young love we were quite sure any plans we made would happen. What could stop them? Now life had shown us otherwise and I was joyful upon receiving a call from a friend saying she had heard there were infants available from our county agency. Infants that were considered hard to place because they were of mixed heritage. We didn't care what their racial background was. If they needed us, we needed them. And so our first call was placed to our county's adoptive services and the process began. We had no idea what was in store for us. Interviews. Separate. Together. Multiple interviews. There were background checks, both personal and financial. They contacted our friends and families, questioning and probing. We had meetings with the workers to discuss our upbringings. We had serious meetings to discuss our feelings about race and how we would deal with a child with a different racial background. We also had physicals to be sure we were healthy enough to parent another child. Young and strong, of course we passed the physicals but we also discovered I was pregnant again. That was not a problem. If I carried this baby to term and we received an infant from the agency, we would be doubly blessed.

We resented not one bit of this home study. If this was necessary to receive the greatest gift we would ever be given, then it was fine. In fact we sometimes laughed and thought perhaps all prospective parents should go through the same screening, not just adoptive ones. The case workers were pleasant, though serious, and we welcomed them.

One of the last steps was a final check through the house to make sure of adequate space for an additional child. I was panicked that if my house was not perfect, we would not be approved. Three days before that inspection I again miscarried. I was nine weeks pregnant. I think that the sadness would have overwhelmed me if I hadn't had the prospect of the other child we were expecting. One delivered by social workers from the county agency. A gift from God, like all children. Friends showed their love and concern by coming and cleaning my already clean house. Calming my fears that if my floors hadn't been washed the night before I would lose this child too.

So, into my spotless house the social workers came. Two of them. They looked at the room we planned to use for the baby and sat down in the living room to chat. I couldn't believe it. My whole house was perfect and I was determined that they would see it all. They did. They laughed, but they did, assuring me that the house was just fine. I wasn't entirely convinced that my new bedspread and spotless floors weren't what had swayed them but I didn't care what it was. We were approved and that was all that mattered.

Now we waited. There were several baby boys ready for placement. No girls. There was also a twenty month old child but the social workers felt the babies would be best for us and they were considering another placement for the toddler. So they checked records, met, and discussed which baby would become ours. They announced that they had picked a child they believed would best fit into the family. A child who was healthy, because they felt another child with problems would be asking too much of us. They told us the child would be placed with us in about a week.

Hearing this news, John and I decided we would take a vacation with Jennica to spend some special time with just her before our new baby boy arrived. Off we went to Florida. Jennica loved it there, enjoying the warm weather and swimming in the hotel's pool but she developed an ear infection and we had to visit the local emergency room. She was ill, weak, and running a fever, when we carried her in. The hospital nurse asked us about her, saying something about her having Down Syndrome. She didn't of course, but they had simply seen her low muscle tone and made a bad diagnosis. I spent the rest of the vacation in our hotel room with a sick child, feeling a combination of anger and despair at the words of the hospital nurse. It wasn't that they had labeled her, or what the label was. It was that even on a vacation, even during the happiest of times, there were reminders that our child was disabled. It was not the trip we had planned but we were learning that few things would be as we planned.

With our time in Florida over and with Jennica feeling a little better, we headed back home. Home to our new baby. His room was waiting for him. It had the blue checkered curtains I had made. Animals and alphabet letters brightly covered one wall. Folded over the side of his crib was a blue and white baby blanket that I had crocheted. We were ready. And then the impossible happened. We received a phone call from our caseworker telling us that the child we were adopting was in the hospital. He had been admitted because of a respiratory infection but while he was there it was discovered that he had cerebral palsy. How could this be? The worker struggled to tell us about this child's problems and also to tell us that he couldn't be placed with us because of them. They would not give us another child who had disabilities. We cried that he was ours, no matter what his condition, but they would not waiver. It was an overwhelming time and it was difficult not to feel despair over the situation.

But a window opened then. Bringing the fresh air of hope. The toddler that we thought had been placed was now available and he was offered to us. Twenty-two months old. Biracial, and if his picture was accurate, beautiful. We headed to our favorite clothing store and celebrated by buying outfits, pajamas, jackets, and little boy socks with rings of different colors circling the tops. We were beyond excited and happy and Jennica was happy with us. She was finally going to have a little brother and she was going to hug and kiss him every time she could catch him.

It was springtime when we became a family of four. The yard was full of blossoms on the many flowering trees. The air was sweet and new and the happiness we felt having a new child was equally sweet. He was a striking little boy. Long curly black hair. Huge black eyes under dark brows. Carmel colored skin, and the prettiest smile ever. It flashed across his face when I brought out the brownies I had baked for this occasion. Jennie smiled back at him and introduced him to our yard. Soon they were running around like the brother and sister that they were meant to be. We named him Joshua but to Jennica he was simply "my brother".

I remember how content we were back then. We

had a delightful son that filled the empty spot in our hearts. We loved watching him run and play. We marveled at him riding a tricycle before he turned two, remembering that Jennica had been over three when she mastered that skill. I woke to him singing in his crib each morning and ran to pick him up, eager to begin another day with him. Jennica was an early riser too, so mornings started early at our house. Days were long and busy then. Setting up a new swing set. Going for walks. Driving to restaurants or parks. We had a perfect family of four. It was an easy time and we found ourselves smiling at how right it felt. People would stop and ask my husband, who has dark coloring, if he had the same curls my son did when he was little. Or they would simply state how much Joshua looked like him. It pleased my husband and confirmed our feeling that this was God's plan.

Jennica was thrilled with her new brother and playmate, but no more than he was with her. We laughed as he followed her around, copying every move she made. Repeating each thing she said. It was a sign of things to come. He adored his sister and was proud of what she did and was. It was cute when he was two and later in life it was admirable.

Having a child who has disabilities makes you keenly aware of development. It makes you applaud and cheer for every skill gained by that child and it makes you stand in awe of children who reach these same milestones easily. It deepens your appreciation for everything that goes right in a child. And so we cheered Jennie on and we celebrated every talent we saw in Joshua. The way they enjoyed each other's company was a beautiful thing and one we marveled at each day.

Jennica went to a regular preschool when she was three. It benefited her by giving her a chance to socialize with children her age and to expose her to different experiences that I couldn't offer at home. In some areas she did well. She quickly learned her colors and knew her shapes and the names of animals. She loved being around the children at the school but some things were reminders that she had problems. Some of the children were uncomfortable around her and didn't want to play. New situations were upsetting for her and left her in tears. She found some of the physical activities impossible and that was frustrating for her and for us too. The teachers were kind, but honest, with both their assessment and their suggestions for Jennie. At the end of the year, while they said they would welcome her back, they hoped we could find a program that was a better fit for her. One that would offer therapy and more intense educational services.

It was a hard thing to accept. We wanted so badly to believe that she was only mildly delayed and that it was going to be okay somehow. I wanted to convince myself that these people were ignorant. I knew they were right but I didn't want them to be. I just wanted my daughter to be an average child. A child without the struggles she faced each day.

There had been another health problem surface the year she turned three. It started on a pleasant day at a special lunch. I had taken Jennica out to eat after her preschool and later we planned on going shopping . Both of these things were treats for her and we were enjoying ourselves, sitting in a booth, eating and chatting. I remember looking at her pretty little face, her brown hair captured in two long braids and her big brown eyes looking intently at me. And then her eyes did something that made my heart stop. Literally. It stopped as fear clenched it. Before I could think, my heart did. Jennica's eyes rolled up. Just a little. She stopped talking. Time stood still. Then just as quickly she finished what she was saying and her eyes were again two pretty brown pools. I tried so hard to act calmly. I didn't want to frighten her. I didn't want her to see the fear that had completely taken over my body. I took a deep breath and we finished our lunch. We went shopping, continuing our day as we had planned. I smiled and laughed and from somewhere far above I watched us, amazed that I could still function.

I went home that night and told my husband. I told him I was concerned it was a seizure. I told him through my tears. I'm not sure if he believed me but it was understandable if he didn't. We had been concerned she would have them from the birth trauma but other than one febrile seizure at about six months old, she had been seizure free. This was so tiny. Her eyes. He hadn't seen it and so it was easy to dismiss. I wish I had been so lucky.

That was the beginning. She was indeed having a type of seizures that they called "minor motor". She was referred to a neurologist. She was sent for tests. EEG's, which terrified her. They didn't hurt her but she hated lying still and having all the leads attached to her head. They tried to give her medication to relax her but being the fighter she was, it only made her groggy. It was a struggle. The test showed nothing. Ridiculous of course, because she didn't have "nothing", she had seizures. The new doctor was a cold and distant man. He refused to really look at or talk to Jennica. He addressed all questions and comments to us. Our visits were frequent because he was not able to control the episodes. Drugs and more drugs were tried. None were effective.

Enter Valproic Acid, a drug from England that was being used for small seizures. It had been used successfully there and, the doctors in England felt it was safe. Desperate to stop the ever increasing seizures, we agreed to enter her into a study being conducted in the United States. In return she would be able to obtain the medicine that was not on the market here. What option was there? Allow the seizures to continue or hope that this new drug was the answer and let the medical profession take our little girl into their world. With a prayer, we agreed.

No small child should have to endure what she did. She had scans and more scans. They injected radioactive material into her veins to help examine her brain. She had more EEG's. She had constant blood work to assure the doctors she was not being hurt by the drug. She could not have aspirin. She could not have orange juice. Sometimes it seemed she could not have a pain free day. She cried and fought each blood test. Each scan. And then one day at the end of the study there were complications from yet another scan. It all became too much for her and for us watching her. We withdrew her from what had become torture. She could still receive the Valproic Acid but we would not allow her to be a test subject any longer. The drug was approved by the FDA shortly after she withdrew and became available to patients in this country, so I'd like to think that her suffering helped another child. It is the only thing that would make what she experienced acceptable. That was Jennica's third year of life. Pre-school and a drug study.

At four, this was behind her and she was enjoying her new brother and a new school. We had located a private school for children with many types of disabilities. Children with autism, Down's syndrome, mild to moderate retardation, and children like Jennica, who didn't fit neatly into a category. It was a long ride every day but it was worth it. Each day I packed up Jennica and Joshua and we headed to the city where the school was located. About forty-five minutes each way.

It was a wonderful facility. Each class had two way mirrors that enabled parents to watch their children engage in different activities. This sometimes brought us a chance to laugh. One day I was watching Jennica being given an IQ test by their psychologist. She was using the Peabody Picture test and on each page there were four pictures that Jennie would look at. The psychologist said a word and had Jennie point to the correct picture. One of the items was an iron. I hate ironing and at that point in my life it was permanent press clothing or I didn't purchase it. Of course my daughter didn't recognize the iron and lost points because of it! I had to laugh and I introduced Jennie to an iron! Another time involved John. He was visiting and watching the students in Jennica's class preparing Apple Crisp. Behind the two way mirror he watched the children happily working. Peeling apples, adding sugar and flour, stirring and smiling. He also observed them wiping their noses and then putting their hands back in the dessert! He was chuckling and enjoying the scene until the teacher stepped out and invited him to join them in eating the freshly baked Apple Crisp. He ate it but he told me it was surely an act of love.

The teachers were young, caring, and knowledgeable. I spent part of my time learning more about Jennica by observing her and part of my time getting to know other mothers who also waited there. As helpful as the school was for Jennica, my time with other parents was equally so. Having a child with a disability is a lonely thing. The world seems to be full of perfect, healthy children. It's a world where you don't really belong. It's a world that sometimes makes you jealous, hurt, or even angry. You love your child but with that love comes pain; for your child and for yourself. You put on your best smile, your cloak of acceptance, your aura of strength, and you walk in the world among your old dreams. It's exhausting, and to be sitting with other mothers who understand is a sweet gift. They know your life. They know your pain. So we all shared as we told our stories. We let our guard down and we cried. We laughed too but it was from the joy of being understood. When you told how happy you were that your child had reached a goal, they knew that happiness. They knew the fierce protective love you had for your child. It was a healing time. A time I gathered both knowledge, strength, and hope. And sometimes I learned a lesson.

Jennica wanted to dance. She wanted to wear ballet shoes with leotards. She wanted to move to the music. She wanted dance lessons. Ridiculous I thought. She didn't walk till she was two. Her muscles were not like those of her peers. And so I told her no. Well, until a wise mother from the school shamed me. She looked me in the eye and told me that if my daughter was capable of asking for dance classes, she should be able to attend dance classes. So what if she couldn't dance like the other children. If she felt like dancing, she should dance. Lesson learned, I signed her up for dance classes. I simply explained her condition to the teachers and then I let her live her dream. Until she was fifteen she danced each year in a recital and she loved every moment of it. Every costume. Every performance. Every little bit of applause. And she had this happiness because a brave mother told me not to be another roadblock in my daughter's life. Bless her.

Everyone at Jennie's school loved my beautiful son. They talked to him and often coaxed him off my lap and onto theirs. Some had younger children his age and he had playmates each day he accompanied me. He and Jennica sat in their car seats in the back of my Beetle as we made that daily trip. So many trips to and from that school but it was our routine. Just the three of us.

Well, just the three of us until something new and wonderful happened. God, with the help of some loving social workers, brought us a little girl. Three months old. Chubby with only a wisp of hair and sweet full cheeks. She too was biracial. Black. White. Beautiful. Ours. We had applied nine months before. Perfect timing we thought. Jennica and Joshua fell in love with her the same way we did. With one look. With one wave of her little fist. With one dimpled smile. We were all overjoyed with our new daughter and sister. Jonna, named for her father.

Jennie loved being with her, bringing me diapers or fresh clothes. She loved helping to feed her and bathe her. She loved her so much she decided Jonna should be her next "Show and Tell" at her school.

The day came when she was picked to share and we marched proudly into the little gym where all the students sat in a circle. When they saw Jennica's little sister they all grinned. They all wanted to be close to her as Jennie and I walked around that circle of love and let each and every child touch Jonna. Jennica's face was beaming with pride and love as she shared her little sister. I suspect that my face was wearing an identical smile. A smile reflecting both my daughter's happiness, and my pleasure in holding my new baby.

Now the four of us drove to the city each day and my new friends fussed over both of my younger children. It was a busy time, but having Jonna made it a sweet time. Jennica was not just attending her special school but she was also going to the local school's kindergarten. I had enrolled her on the recommendation of her special preschool teachers. They felt that she was ready but that she would benefit from a full day of stimulation. At that time kindergarten was a half day program, so mornings she worked with specialists and in the afternoon she went to kindergarten. She was excited to be with new children and I was happy for her. Unfortunately we soon realized that it was not going to be a completely positive experience.

School and Heartache

Every day, after a quick lunch, I would pull up to the little annex where the kindergarten was housed. The sidewalk leading to Jennica's room was about thirty feet long, and there her teacher would stand at the door greeting her students. One day I watched my little girl walk her unique and sweetly awkward walk to a class she adored and a teacher she loved. Her shiny brown hair was in two ponytails, garnished with pretty white ribbons. They bounced with each step she took as she swung her book bag, so proud to be a student. I was proud too. Proud of her progress and her strength. I loved watching her from the car and I thought she looked adorable in her saddle shoes and blue plaid dress. I made that dress, sewing each stitch with gratitude that she was going to be able to attend this neighborhood school. That she had reached this important milestone. It was a pretty picture. My little ones in the back seat, me smiling in the front seat, and Jennica eagerly approaching her class.

I saw a little boy running up to the annex and I wondered if he was in Jennica's class. I didn't recognized him so I thought perhaps he was in the other kindergarten room housed there. I was thinking he was cute with short sandy hair and obviously a lot of energy as he bounded to his class. And then he stopped. He stopped as he passed Jennie. He turned around, he looked at her, and he spit in her face. I was stunned and for a moment I sat there. Frozen with both anger and surprise. Jennie continued into her class and then they were both gone. I had two small children in the car but out they came and together we headed to the school's office. I was livid and I'm sure that was apparent as I entered the school. I was certain the administration would be shocked too but that belief was short lived.

Let's just say that from that moment on I realized Jennica was not welcome there. That she was a nuisance, a puzzle, and that the place she adored was only meant for children like the healthy little boy who recognized her for what she was. Different. There was no support from the school's administration. There was no outrage or sympathy. There was only a cold breeze ushering in Jennica's future at that school.

And so the battle began. The administration wanted her gone. We discovered that it was their policy to ship all children with physical disabilities to another school north of the city. Attending the school would involve a forty-five minute bus ride each way. It was a school that served children with visual and hearing impairments. Children who used wheelchairs. Children that had multiple and severe challenges. There were children there that Jennica's school did not want. While Jennie's issues were not as severe as most of these children, she did have multiple handicaps and so her school determined that she belonged at this other location. As her parents, we felt she belonged with the neighborhood kids. She tested in the normal range of intelligence and was able to be self sufficient at school. To send her on a bus ride each day for an hour and a half seemed ridiculous. That was time that had a hundred better uses.

The school began to call meetings. First small ones with limited personnel. They extolled the virtues of the distant school. They discussed and dissected Jennica's condition. What they would not do is listen to our concerns about the bus ride or the negative impact of Jennica not attending her local school. So the meetings continued and escalated. Meeting after meeting until the final attack when they lined up eleven people hoping that the show of force would make us retreat. That was a difficult day. John and I sitting there with eleven people and their "professional opinions" telling us once again that Jennie could not attend their school. I remember going home that afternoon feeling both anger and sadness. Wondering why I could not find support for my daughter whom I believed to be capable of learning at this school. After the tears I went to work and began to assemble my own team of experts.

First, I called the local Special Education Resource Center and explained the situation. They are an impartial agency that offers support and help to children who have disabilities and to those who work with these children. They arranged to test Jennica and determine what they thought the best course of action would be. Then I called her pediatrician who was horrified that we were encountering this kind of resistance from Jennica's school. The doctor contacted her school and assured the administration that there was no medical reason for her not to attend her local school. He praised her spirit and her intelligence and he made it clear that he was unhappy over her treatment. The SERC center, after testing and observing Jennica in her kindergarten class, strongly recommended to us that Jennie stay in her local school district. With these people behind us we attended one more meeting.

We went feeling confident that we were fighting for what was best for our daughter. Having other people there to support us gave us courage to face these people again, but even with this newfound courage my heart raced and my mouth was dry. I was determined not to cry but worried that tears would come unbidden. When the school staff began explaining to the SERC personnel why Jennica couldn't attend their school, the SERC psychologist sat straight up in her chair and looked directly at the principal. With a clear and steady voice she said that any six year old with the intelligence and perception to distinguish the color "butterscotch" should be in a regular class. She had previously gone over her testing results and with this final statement the room became quiet. There was nothing left to be said. Jennica was going to attend this school for first grade.

Battles are not something I enjoy. Not then. Not now. But the situation with Jennica's school made me stronger. I learned that I had the strength to challenge obstacles in my daughter's way. I never learned to enjoy conflict, and I chose my battles, but I had the courage to fight for what I believed was right. Having a child with disabilities will change you. It can crush you or it can make you aware of strength buried deep within you. Jennie's school situation hurt me and frustrated me but ultimately it made me grow. The love I had for my daughter made me strong.

Jennica never knew of this struggle and when she

headed off to her first grade classroom she took it for granted that this was the next step in her life. That she would be greeted happily by people who welcomed her, and in some ways she was. Her regular education teacher was cool to her, to the idea of having her for a student, but she was never cruel. The parents of her classmates were friendly to me and some told me how pleased they were to have Jennie in their child's class. One parent shared with me that because of my battle the previous spring, their child, like Jennica, was receiving O.T., and attending the school. I later became friends with this woman and was happy that we had been able to help her and her child. Jennica went to a Learning Disabilities classroom for additional help and her teacher there was kind and hard working. Jennie enjoyed going to her class and didn't mind that it was in an old storage closet. No windows. Six feet across and perhaps twelve feet deep. She didn't mind because she was welcome there and that feeling makes almost any setting acceptable. I do believe, however, that having a L. D. class in a closet spoke loudly about this school's view of children with challenges. About their desire to serve them. All in all, the year was uneventful and we were able to focus on other parts of our life.

Life at Seven

Thankfully there were lots of other parts. The summer before Jennica began first grade we bought a bigger house in the same area. Each child had their own room and lots of places to play, though most of the playing that summer centered around the backyard pool. It was perfect for Jennica with her cerebral palsy, giving her a place to feel free and happy. It did the same for our other children who would have gladly spent all day there if they were allowed. Joshua learned to swim and Jonna drifted around in her baby float turning her curly light brown hair to blond. They were all sweet water babies and I was their happy mother.

I returned to school that year. I was accepted at a charming private college not too far from our home. I returned to get a degree in teaching children with disabilities and this school offered an excellent program. I had left college when I married John and now seemed to be the right time to finish what I started years before. So, Jennica was in first grade, Joshua was in preschool, and Jonna spent a few hours at a sitter's home, as I studied teaching with a new sense of purpose. As the mother of Jennica, I felt I could bring understanding to parents and a heartfelt dedication to my students.

Jennica had a lot going on in her life that year. Besides school she had her dance classes, which she continued to adore, and a new activity called Indian Princesses. This was a YMCA sponsored group for fathers and daughters that promoted strong, long term relationships. I sewed costumes for both of them. A vest with beads for John and a Indian princess dress for Jennica. They added headbands and moccasins, which they made themselves. Thus attired, they headed off each Tuesday night to join eight other sets of fathers and daughters. They met at different houses, played games, went on field trips, and even camped out. They both loved it, enjoying the extra time they spent together. One night was extra special and touched my husband's heart deeply.

It was a magical night. A father, daughter, dance. I bought Jennica a new dress and new shiny patent leather shoes. Her father put on a suit and a smile and off they headed for a night of fun with their tribal friends. Jennica was ready to dance the night away in her own special seven year old style. And dance they did. That would have been enough but there was more: there was a dance contest, with a purse and wallet for prizes, and Jennica was beyond excited about it. Her father was a bit more realistic. He knew how much Jennie loved to dance but he also knew there was a room full of pretty little girls that weren't disabled and they too loved to dance. Still they entered and they danced. And then a miracle happened. They won, and in that moment all the goodness that can exist in people covered my sweet daughter and her father. When they came home Jennica carried her new leather purse and her father his new wallet, along with a renewed belief in people. To this day his special wallet is safely tucked away in his chest of drawers and the memory of that night in his heart.

Though I wasn't there at the dance, I was there when they returned home and Jennie burst into the house filling it with her happiness. Her belief in herself. Her love for her father. I was there when my husband came in with his heart on his face. Having a child like Jennica brings home too many heartaches but occasionally it brings home a sweet memory that lasts forever. I'd like to believe that the men who gave us this gift were blessed many times over. They deserved it.

There were other sweet memories from that year. Watching the children grow and play was a blessing. To see the love they had for each other never grew old. Three children with different genes who knew that they were brother and sisters and that genes had nothing to do with it. I believed with all my heart that God had brought me each child and that each was truly mine. I watched Joshua race down the sidewalk on his Big Wheel screeching to a sudden stop or waving at me with a happy smile on his face. I watched Jonna unfold baskets of laundry that I had just folded and her smile was just as happy. I watched Jennica's joy at having her brother and sister as they shared their days together and I knew that life, though sometimes a challenge, was good.

I was enjoying my return to college, loving my teachers, and the small pretty campus. I was older than most of the student body but that was fine, everyone was friendly and I was there to learn. I was eager to complete my degree and begin my teaching career. I could see the finish line and I was more focused than I had ever been.

And so the Heavens, recognizing that I was almost comfortable, thought it was time for a new challenge. It came wrapped in an opportunity for John. He had been recruited by a business two hours north of our home. Two hours. How could this work? My feet were planted and my life was finally making some sense, I loved both my school and the fact that I was going to be able to finally finish my degree. I loved my home and my new friends. I had no desire to move and leave the life we had built and I couldn't pretend differently, but John was thrilled with this offer. He wanted it. Me? I couldn't even picture having to find a new pediatrician. Big sigh. Deep breath. We were a family and we were moving.

Moving North

There was one positive. We had a chance to find a school district that would embrace Jennica. One that would support us and work with us. While Jennica **was** in her local school, we could never forget that she wasn't wanted. That she was resented. That we were disliked because we had battled their system. Because we had questioned their policy. Now we could start afresh and explore our options. We decided to set up appointments with three school districts and discuss our unique situation with them. Not only did we have Jennica, we had two biracial children that we wanted to be comfortable and welcomed. Somewhere they could look around a classroom and see other children who looked like them. So, we went looking for the place that would give all our children what they needed. A place our family could be happy.

We had a list of questions and a list of needs. We needed a school district that was racially mixed. We needed a district that was equipped to educate Jennica and help her grow. It was a lot to look for and only one district seemed to offer what we needed. To our surprise they offered it with open arms and we were relieved that we had found acceptance in this new community. It was in a small college town known for it's liberal views and historic significance. It had a racially diverse population and to us it seemed ideal. While I had left so much behind, I began to think this move could be a good thing.

Housing was another problem. We were looking

for houses with as much space as we currently had. There was nothing like that on the market and in the end we bought a smaller fixer upper that had four bedrooms. We closed on this house in August and moved in the week before school started.

It wasn't an easy move. It was one of those hot, muggy August days. Steamy and still. I cleaned the house we were leaving, tears and sweat mixing with the soapy water. I was determined to leave the place spotless, grateful that a friend had bought our home as soon as he knew we were moving. I wanted the house to be fresh and clean. Ready to become his. So, three young children scrambled around as I cleaned, my long hair tied back in an attempt to keep cool. An attempt that failed. Once the movers had packed all of our belongings we climbed into the car and drove off. I cried and felt an overwhelming loss as we pulled away. Tired, dirty, sad, but trying to be hopeful, I headed to our new home town. My husband was tired too, but excited. My children were sleepy and perhaps confused. They were young with Jennica at seven, Joshua five, and Jonna only two but they all said good bye to their home as we left. Happy, sad, tired, confused, no matter what we were feeling, we were on our way to a new life.

We spent that night in a local hotel. We showered and fell into our beds exhausted, both physically and mentally. The hotel's air conditioning was a welcomed relief after the long hot day. Early the next morning we were up and over to our new home where cleaning began again. The former owners had left many belongings in the house and my brothers and parents met us there to help clear things out. We were grateful for their help and their good humor. My brother Bob found a shallow closet at the end of a hallway and pronounced it the "vase closet". They all made fun of a falling down sun room off the side of the house. Three brothers, a bit of kicking and pushing and it was gone. Light flooded into the house, the next door neighbor told us thank you, and our first remodeling was done.

With the house clean and furniture moved in, we took a deep breath and spent a few days becoming familiar with the neighborhood before the beginning of school. The children happily discovered there were many other kids living on the street. One child, who lived directly across from us, brought freshly baked cookies from his mother. He stood there, an adorable carrot top with a welcoming smile, holding the chocolate chip cookies and I remember thinking how sweet it was and how hopeful I was that we could make this neglected house a place where happiness surrounded us.

With Jennica and Joshua off to their new school, Jonna and I had some quiet time at home. Though there were many things that needed to be done there, much of my time was spent feeling sad. The move had destroyed my carefully rebuilt life. My lovely home was gone. My dearly loved college was gone. My friends were left behind. I was discouraged and lonely in this new place. It seemed that I would never finish my degree and teach. I was tired and depressed, and for awhile I simply let life wash over me. I did what I needed to do. I signed Jennica up for dance classes. For speech and occupational therapy. I became acquainted with the town, local shopping, and the children's school. I spent pleasant hours with Jonna. She was only two and it was nice to be able to give her my undivided attention. So we sang and played games and spent a lot of time snuggling. I did all of these things, but inside my mind was thinking and evaluating, and my heart was heavy. Life was feeling difficult and not much like I thought it would be. It was darker, like the new house. It was a time of giving up my personal dreams. Letting them go and considering them frivolous. I didn't know what else to do. It seemed that each time I tried to set goals and work towards them I hit a roadblock, so maybe I was meant to be a good mother and wife. Period. I tried to adjust my thinking and move on.

Of course part of my sadness was Jennica. There was always a struggle going on. Perhaps it was health related or maybe an issue at school. Sometimes it was just grieving. Grieving the loss of a normal life for my daughter. Disabilities do not go away. They are identified. They are worked on or worked around but they don't go away. And the cuteness of a small child becomes an older awkward child with problems. I loved Jennica. I accepted her as she was, but constant daily issues combined with worries for her future gave me little peace. So each day the heavy sad feeling accompanied me as I did my best.

I threw myself into the role of mother and wife. I baked bread, I sewed clothes, I canned and froze food from our little garden and from nearby farms. I fixed big healthy meals every night for my family. I was proud of my hard work and eventually I just gave up my own dreams and dreamed for my family instead. I loved raising my children. Whether I was cooking or sewing for them, or simply singing to them as I bathed them each night, I loved them and loved being their mother. Everything else might have gone "topsy turvy" but that remained the same. They were beautiful, cheerful, children and John and I both loved being with them. We stood together and worked for them, always grateful they were ours and fully appreciating what a gift they were. I think it was partly because we enjoyed parenting and perhaps partly because we felt we had room for one more child, that we decided to adopt again. Whatever the reason, we knew we wanted another child.

It was during this time that I gathered myself together and tried to adjust my attitude. I was determined to make the best of what my life seemed destined to be. The first thing I did was paint my gloomy bedroom a cheery sky blue. It was a declaration of sorts. A symbol that life was good and I would see that good. So out with the gold walls and heavy dark drapes and in with blue walls and fluffy white curtains,

With my improved outlook we set about bringing our next child home. We discussed babies, and though I loved the idea, John was hesitant to return to raising infants. He felt that perhaps we should become parents to an older child that needed a home. I quickly agreed, and soon after that we contacted an agency. The county agency was helpful and friendly. Later we became spokespersons for them, often speaking at meetings about adopting hard to place children. Within a few months we had become parents to an impish ten year old girl, Julie. She had light brown hair, huge blue eyes, and she reminded us of a young Haley Mills. We welcomed her into our lives and we became a family of six. Not a conventional family but certainly one that God had planned and made possible. When we looked over our four beautiful children we knew we had been blessed.

Jennica's first year at her new school had been successful. When we first moved and spoke to the school personnel about her, they had suggested she repeat first grade and begin again in this new atmosphere. We felt it would give her a stronger beginning and so we agreed. They placed her in a classroom where she was blessed with the kindest and most hardworking of teachers. He was determined to help her read and devoted extra time each day working with her, one on one. In addition to her regular classroom she attended a resource room where a talented, tender, special education teacher devoted herself to improving the lives of her students. She was eager to help Jennie and always treated us like we were a part of that plan.

While Jennie seemed to have a gift for being happy in any environment, she thrived at this new school. She made friends and grew in the friendly, accepting atmosphere. She learned to read that year. Her new teachers, using their skills and imaginations, opened the world of books to her. While she had always loved being read to, now she was doing the reading. It was difficult to know who was the most thrilled. Her teachers, her parents, or herself. We were all proud. That I am sure of.

Becoming a Family of Six

There was a little summer left after Julie came to stay. We spent it working out the new family dynamics and also having some fun. Bedrooms had changed. Jonna and Jennie now shared a room. Each had a pretty white bed and matching bedspreads. Jonna had never liked sleeping by herself so she was thrilled. Jennica seemed to welcome Jonna and though there was less room for both of them, they also had companionship. We had given Julie a room by herself. We redecorated the room, making it a soft and sunny yellow, trimmed with white. We filled it with new furniture and hoped it would please her. I think having her own room made it easier for her to adjust to our family. A quiet place of her own. The children had made neighborhood friends by now and spent long days outside, riding bikes, playing on the swing set, and digging holes to China. Our extended families lived in small towns close by and we traveled to see them and introduced our new daughter. They welcomed her as they had welcomed our other children. Perhaps not always understanding our life, but always accepting one more. Of course they weren't the only people who seemed confused about our family. It seemed like there were a lot of others.

We got stared at. That is the truth of it. Most stares weren't hostile, though some were, actually people seemed more puzzled by us. Four children that didn't look alike. It didn't bother John and I, after all we had assembled this tribe and we were quite happy about it, but the children hated it. They complained each time they were looked up and down until finally I declared that it was only because no one had ever seen so many good looking people in one place. It made the children laugh and I often repeated it throughout their childhoods. A sense of humor can help most situations and I knew they would all need to be able to laugh at difficult times in their lives. And I knew there would be difficult times.

That summer we traveled to see a family farm and fed baby calves. We headed to the local amusement park, as we did each and every year, making a long day and night of it and returning home dirty, tired, and happy. We traveled south to see old friends and stay in a hotel where the children could swim. They missed their swimming pool and happily swam for hours. It was there that we discovered that Julie also loved the water. It was a good summer and then it was once again time for school.

I know that many parents are delighted when school opens again. They are ready for their children to have that structure and they look forward to a little more time for themselves. I just didn't happen to be one of those parents. Summer was not only freedom for my children, it was freedom for myself. Freedom from the constant reminder that Jennica struggled. Yes, she made progress. Yes, she had dedicated and pleasant teachers. But still the struggles remained. Even her health concerns escalated during the school year with exposure to classroom germs. And always there was my concern for her happiness and fitting in. Add three other children with their own special academic needs and school was difficult to be excited about. Summer, full of neighborhood children and free time, was easy. The school year often wasn't.

It began whether I was ready or not. The children had new backpacks full of supplies, new shoes, new outfits, and new teachers. Jennica was in the second grade this year. Julie was in the fourth, Joshua in the first, and Jonna began preschool. On the first day of school I lined the children up in front of the house and took their picture, their faces showing the mixture of excitement and apprehension that they felt. Four children scrubbed and ready to start a new school adventure. Then into the car they went so that I could deliver them to their schools.

For the first time in eight years my house was quiet and empty. At first I was a little puzzled about this new free time. I remember taking Jonna to her little school, returning home, sitting on the couch, and thinking, what now? Of course that didn't last long. Her school time was short and there were plenty of household duties to fill those hours. Just in case I couldn't keep busy, I volunteered at Jonna's preschool once a week. She was hesitant about attending, so my being a part of this new school helped. Things were changing and this was both an end and a beginning.

Life was full. Besides raising four children and trying to meet all of their needs, I had to find the extra time to take Jennica to additional speech and occupational therapy twice a week. We were fortunate to have a children's center in a neighboring town that could provide therapy and give me a little guidance too. It made a long day for all of us but there was no choice. She needed the extra help and I was happy we found good people to provide it. Still, it must have been a long day for all of the children and they were relieved to be home when we pulled into our driveway. They would change into old clothes, have a snack, do their homework, and head outside to play for awhile before supper time. I loved to cook for them and they all enjoyed eating what I cooked, so this was a favorite part of our day. John was home for dinner each night and it was a special time for us, looking at each other and around the table of children. This had been our dream and now it was here. We bowed our heads for grace and then ate supper and told about our days. John and I had made ourselves a promise that dinner would be together and it would be stress free for all. We kept that promise and so it was a time when we bonded as a family. A family that we had built and that we treasured.

Jennica was showing improvement in her classroom and that was a relief, but as usual, something else marched in and become a new challenge for her. This year it was seizures and hearing aids. Jennie had been seizure free for several years and her neurologist felt she should try going without the medication she took to prevent them. Months passed with no problem and we became very hopeful. Then one day as she walked out of her physical education class she collapsed to the floor with a grand mal seizure. This was something she had never experienced before and it frightened her as much as it did us. We immediately contacted her doctor who put her back on her medication. For several months she had smaller episodes until the medication was at a therapeutic level. I never again agreed to her going off of it. We eventually reduced the dosage to a very low level but I would not allow her to go through that again.

During the same year her school speech therapist

discovered that she had a hearing loss. It had not been detected before and we were almost reluctant to believe she had one more disability to deal with. Off to the ENT she went and there the loss was confirmed. Not kindly confirmed either. The specialist was furious that this had not been discovered until now. He yelled and scowled at us as if we had somehow neglected her. No matter how many doctors and speech therapists she had seen over the years. No matter how carefully everyone had followed her health issues. We were to blame. We felt terrible. Not guilty really, we knew what had been done previously, but so sad for her, and honestly, angry at the doctor's manner. It was determined that she would need just one aid. It was ordered, and shortly thereafter she had a small, flesh colored aid that fit into her ear.

She hated it from the first. She was aware of all the differences already present between her classmates and herself, and she was angry about having one more. She would take it out while at school or she would put her hand up by it to make it scream from the feedback. I guess she felt that was at least entertaining and her classmates would be amused. We tried to encourage her to wear it, comparing it to wearing glasses and by explaining it's importance, but she never accepted it and by the time she was a teenager she had won. She could hear well enough without it and she was done. We won the battle but she won the war.

Her grandparents were as dismayed as we were when they learned about her hearing loss. My parents accepted it as John and I did. John's mother did the same, but his father was devastated and told us he would not even talk about it, let alone look at it. It seemed to be more than he could handle. Perhaps it was because it was an outward and visible sign of his granddaughter's problems. I was startled by his reaction and again realized how Jennica's disabilities had affected all of her family. We on a deeper level, but all of her family had at least a kernel of sadness in their hearts because of the problems she had to face. It was possible for her grandfather to deny this situation and though I wish he handled it differently, it was his right. I couldn't of course. I couldn't escape anymore than Jennica could. Her problems were always with me. I was always trying to find solutions to help or least to distract her from her disabilities. Lying in bed at night I would go over and over current problems, making sleep elusive and most often solving nothing. When I could make things better for her, I made things better for myself. I could watch her struggle less and therefore I struggled less too. As long as I was helping, I was strong but each time a new problem surfaced or a new hurt was revealed, I was wounded. I was without breath, sick with sadness. There was no protection from this hurt. Not for her, nor for me. Her pain was immediate and mine was mingled with fears for her future.

Of course Jennica did have pleasure in her life, along with the problems. She had dance classes, Brownies, and art classes. She had neighborhood playmates and a family that adored her. She had a wonderful summer camp for children with disabilities that she attended each summer. She also had a cat named Rosie. We were not looking for another pet but one day Jennica was visiting a friend from dance class and while she was there she was introduced to a litter of kittens. One tiger cat, the smallest of the litter, looked up at Jennie and stole her heart. She called me and asked if she could be the mother to this cat. What could I possibly say to that plea? We already had a dog and a cat but this would be her cat. Jennie loved her fiercely from the first and Rosie loved her back. Rosie was always there for her and I never regretted bringing her home. She was one of Jennica's childhood pleasures and she was her faithful friend.

It was during this time that Jennica decided she wanted to join a local children's choir. It was a small group and some children from our church and Jennie's school belonged. I wasn't concerned nor surprised. Jennie had always loved music and though her voice was affected by her cerebral palsy, I didn't think it would matter. These were children, not a professional group. The director had Jennie audition and refused to accept her. I was more shocked than angry but when the woman then tried to recruit her sister, Julie, I was disappointed that anyone would be so unfeeling. Julie was even more angry than I was and told the director that if her sister wasn't good enough then she wasn't either! Of course I was proud of Julie but I was disheartened by the insensitivity of this woman. Jennica was hurt. Hurt and handicapped, but I doubt as handicapped as the choir director. After all, Jennie had a heart.

That year brought problems but it also brought a healing vacation to Disney World. Jennica was thrilled and her brother and sisters were right there with her. We planned the trip for their spring vacation and rented a motor home, thinking it would be easier and more economical. In addition to our four children we invited the young girl, who babysat for them each Saturday night, to join us. We thought she would enjoy it and that she could relieve us from time to time. So, we all planned and packed and lived in anticipation for our trip to Florida and it was a nice way to distract ourselves.

We had taken Jennica and Joshua to Disney World when she was four years old. My parents had joined us in a rented RV and together we had explored campgrounds and beaches in Florida. Now, as experienced campers we set out once again for the magic of Disney and the warmth of the south. The children were excited and eager for this adventure. John was ready to be the captain of our motor home and I was looking forward to the sunshine and simple fun of being on a family trip. Off to Florida we went. We stayed in the same campground we had stayed in years before when we had traveled there with their grandparents. It was a pretty place with lots of Spanish moss hanging from the plentiful shade trees. There were friendly people there. Some pedaling around on bicycles, waving and smiling, happy to have us join them. There was also a beautiful pool for the children to play in and sometimes for us to join in. It was pure pleasure to see their upturned faces as they floated around in the sunshine looking as happy as children should look.

Like our winter coats and our heavy boots, we shed our troubles and our stress. We left them back North as we played in the swimming pool, on warm sandy beaches, and as we wandered through the streets of Disney World. We even celebrated Easter in Florida. Bringing the children's' baskets, and all the goodies to fill them with, was a challenge, but it was worth it when they woke up in our little camper and discovered that the Easter Bunny had found them in Florida! We returned sunburned but happy, renewed for whatever fate would dish up. Jennica and her siblings had had a chance to simply be children and happy ones at that. What more could I ask for.

Peaceful Times and Personal Changes

Sometimes there is a lull in life and this was ours. While challenges remained a daily occurrence, they were smaller ones. Ones I could deal with without lying awake at night. It was a time to breath and look around a little. A time to think about what to focus on next. Not in a studied and deliberate way, more like a walking around, the pots on the back burner type of thinking. I think mothers are good at that and I was no exception. Anyway, one day at a dance rehearsal I was sitting next to another dance mommy and as we were dressing our girls in their pretty costumes, we got to talking. She told me that she was going back to school and that the local community college had partnered with a university that had a strong education program. She was excited because she didn't have to drive a long distance to finish up her teaching degree. I perked up. Yes, I know I said I gave up my personal dreams but I guess I had just put them on hold. Before I knew it, she had convinced me to enroll in school and finish this degree once and for all. The dance recital was lovely. Jennica and Julie both danced on the big stage with lots of family watching and cheering. I was clapping as madly as all the others but in my mind I was taking that pot off the back burner and beginning to stir it.

I enrolled. The ease my friend had emphasized didn't apply to me because of my special education major and after one semester at the local community college I had to drive an hour each day to the university. I wasn't happy about that and I was worried about how I would handle four children, therapy, homework, and household tasks, but I was going to do it. The first semester was doable but it soon became apparent that when I had to drive to the university I was going to need some help. I was taking a heavy load, over twenty credit hours a term, and besides the driving, the class time, the school observation time, I had homework. Lots of it. I wasn't sure I could do it until John stepped in. His job required frequent travel which further complicated this situation. He changed positions at his company to a job that kept him home and offered him more flexibility. He learned to braid hair, cook dinners, keep the children organized, and simply do what I couldn't. It was a gift and I couldn't have done it without him. I barely made it with him. I would stay up late doing homework along with laundry and cleaning, until I couldn't think clearly anymore and then begin again the next morning at five, when the house was quiet. For a year and a half this was my routine. I was focused. I was driven. When I wasn't picturing myself in my own classroom, I was picturing myself driving a minivan. Yes, a minivan! If you have four children a van is a mother's dream. Believe me! Finally, on a beautiful June day, I walked across the stage and received my diploma. My children, dressed in their Sunday best, were watching. My parents were watching. My husband was watching and I am almost certain I heard him breath a sigh of relief. I got my first job as a tutor in a nearby school system. I was delighted to be on my way and was even happier when I was hired a few months later by our town's schools. I was with my children, doing what I had dreamed of, and yes, I was driving a minivan!

I hope I was an inspiration for my children. I know for certain that Jennica inspired me. She worked so hard with what she was given that I knew I should do the same. I know Jennie and my other children were proud that their mom was a teacher and I was determined to do my best. I was determined to give other children what my daughter had been given, and more.

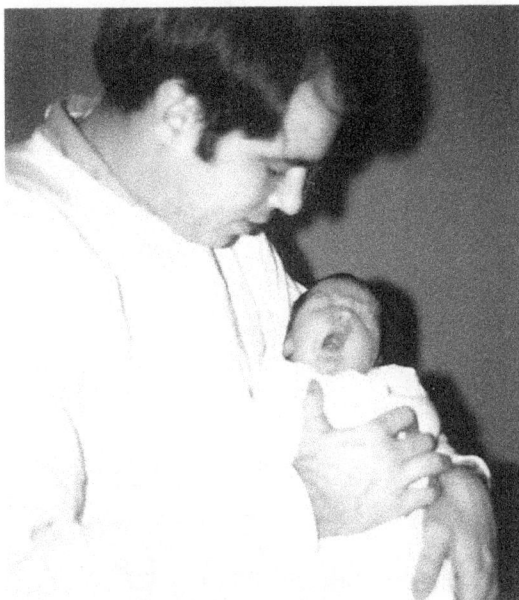

Proud new Daddy

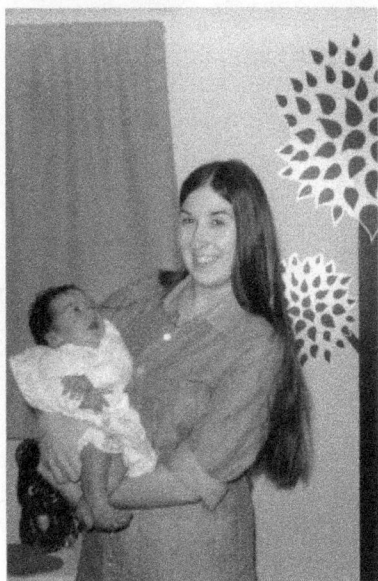

First day at home

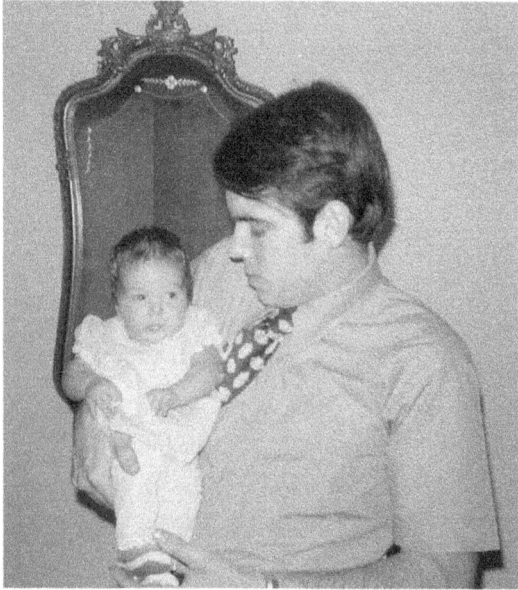

Ready for an outing

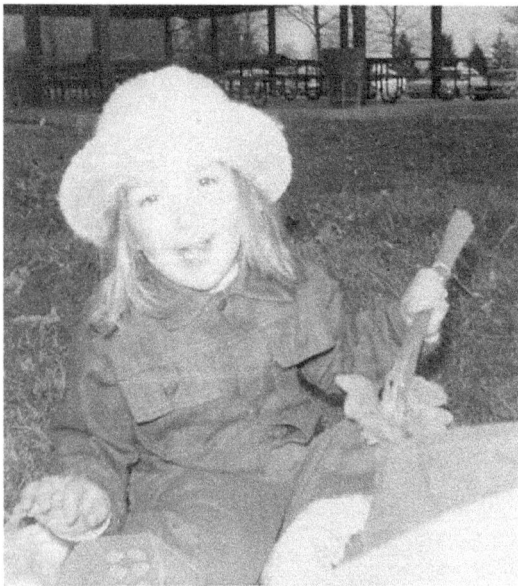

A day at the park.

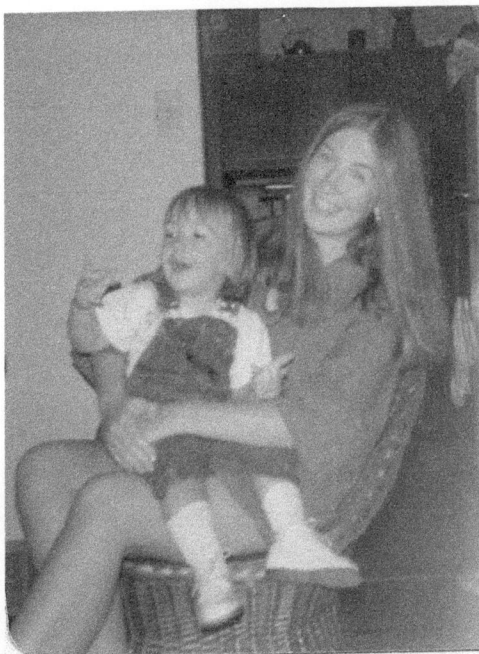

John says we're his two beauties.

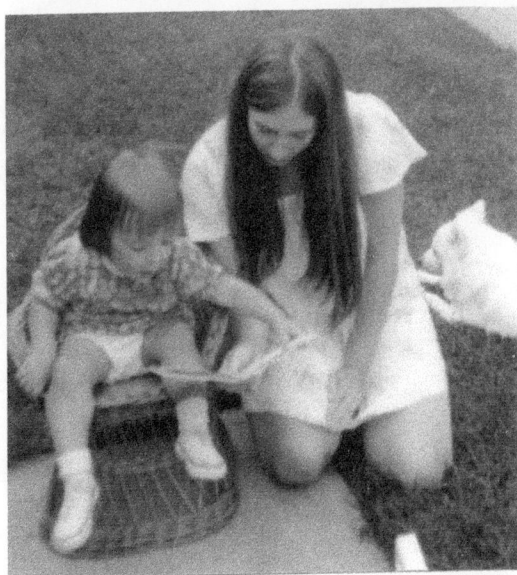

Enjoying a summer day with Mom and Yukie.

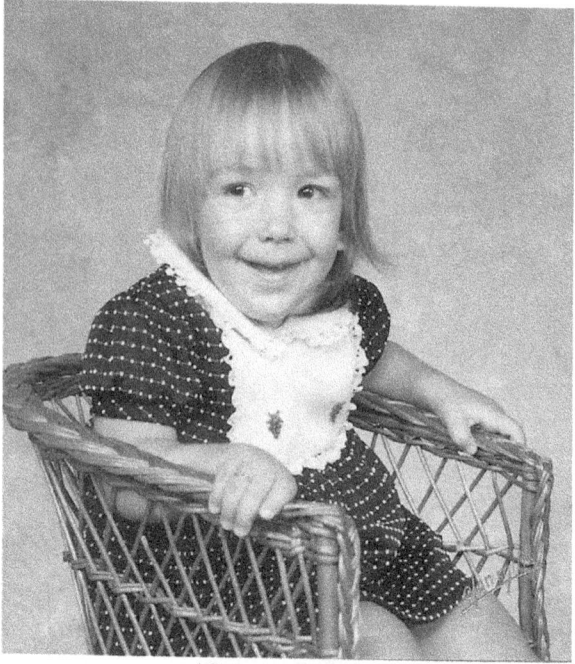

Always smiling

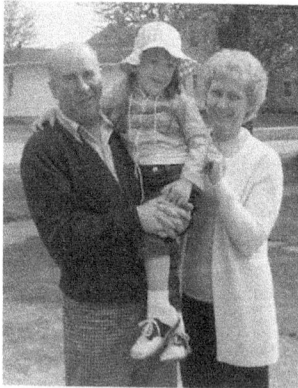

With Grandpa and Grandma Johnson

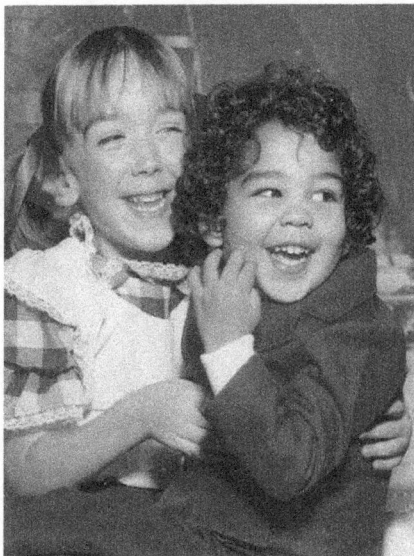

A new brother, Joshua

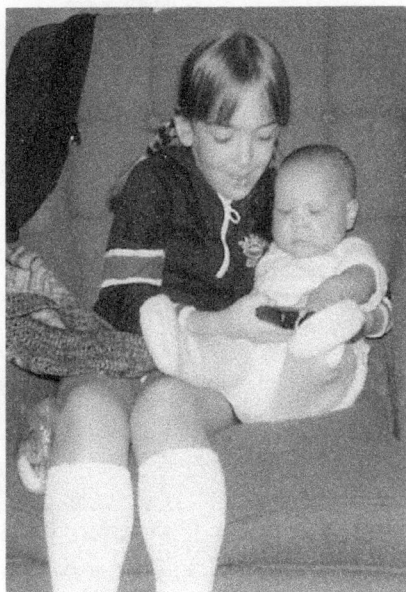

With her baby sister, Jonna

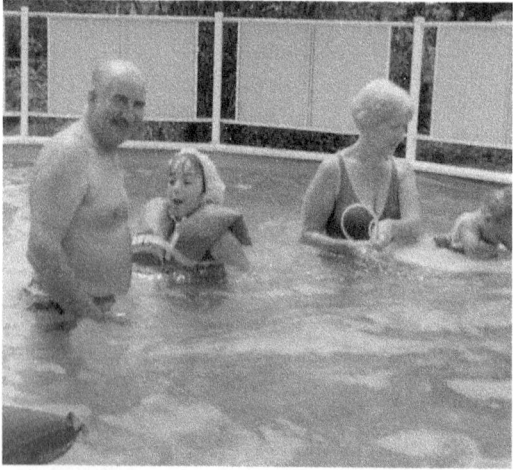

Enjoying our backyard pool with Grandpa and Grandma Johnson.

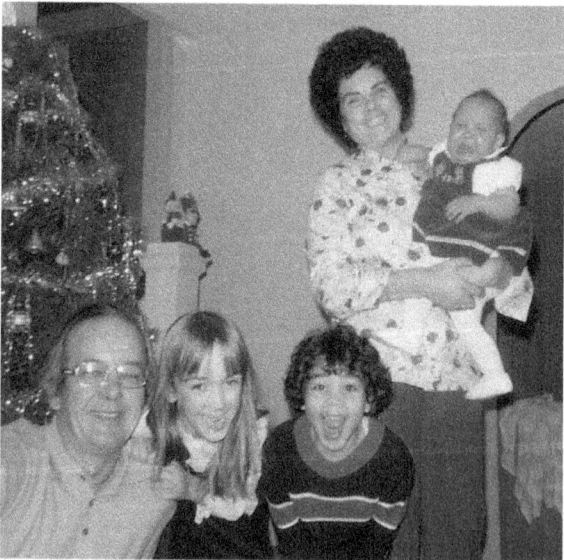

Mostly a Merry Christmas with Grandpa and Grandma Thonen.

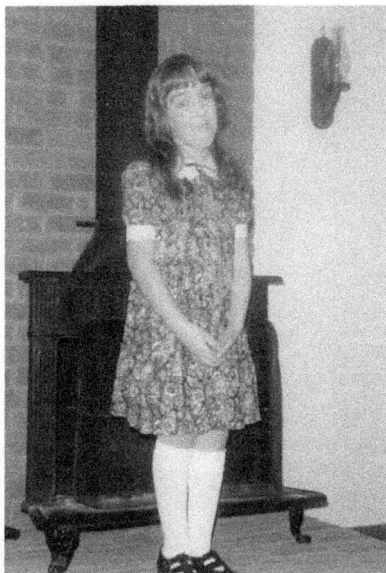

Ready for the Indian Princess dance.

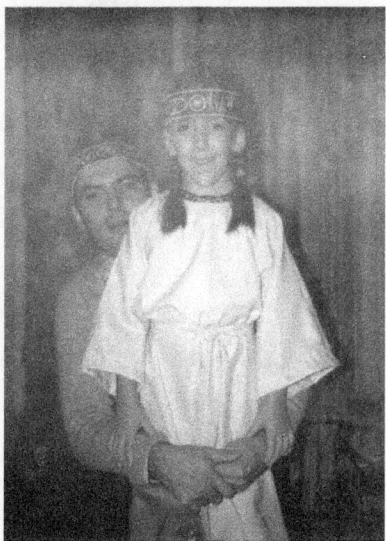

Jen and Dad in Indian Princess costumes.

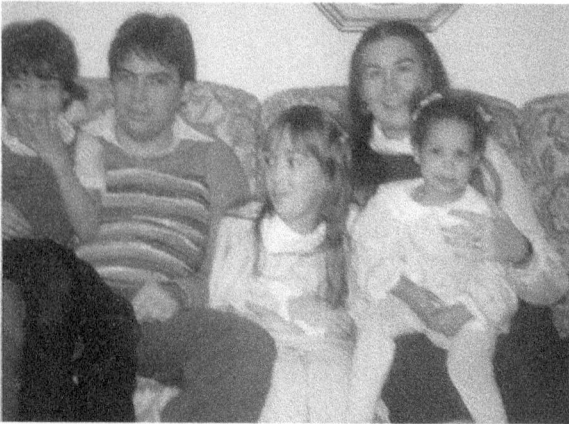

Visiting at Grandpa and Grandma Johnson's house.

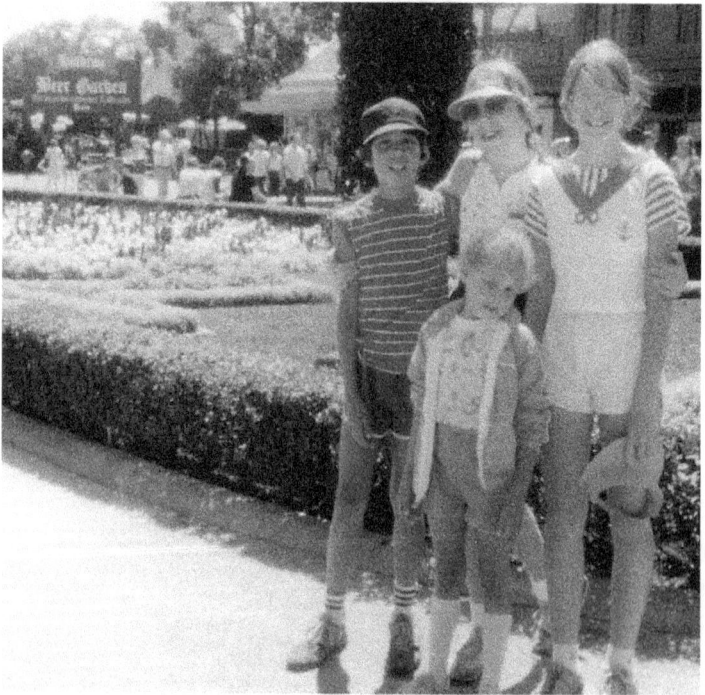

A day at the amusement park.

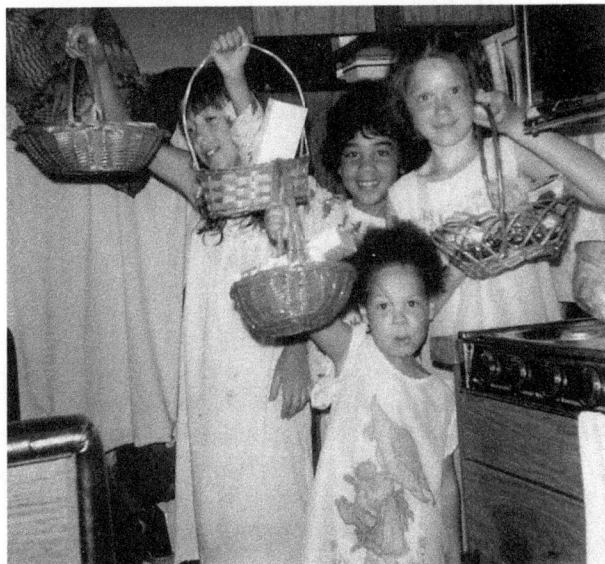

The Easter Bunny visited our vacation camper.

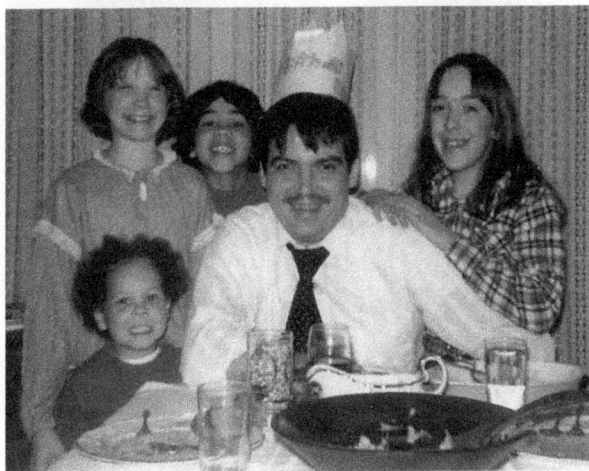

Birthday celebration

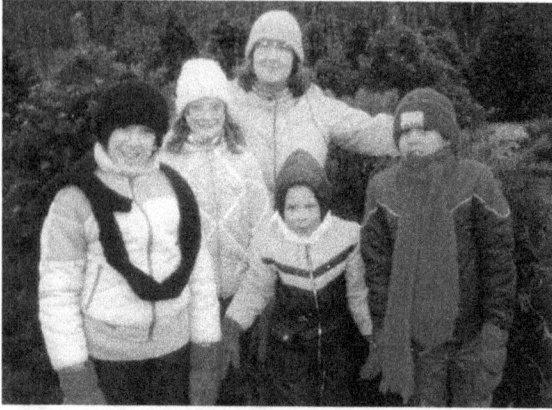

Our annual quest for the perfect Christmas tree.

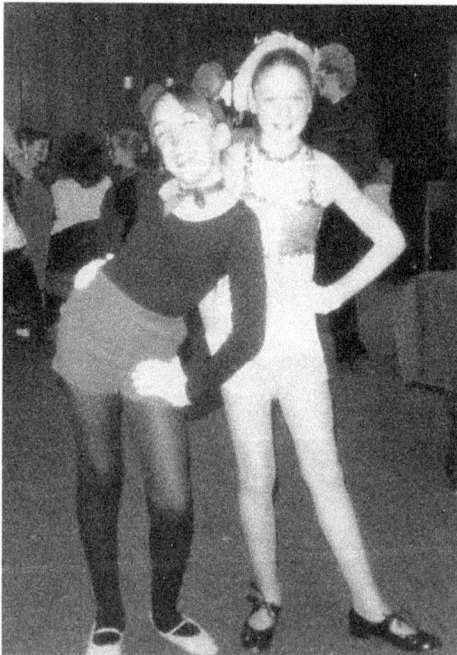

Backstage at the dance recital

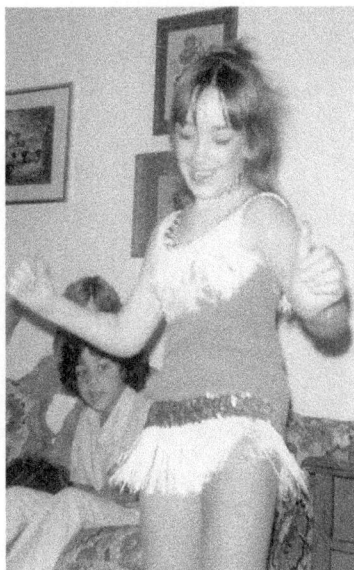

Love to dance!

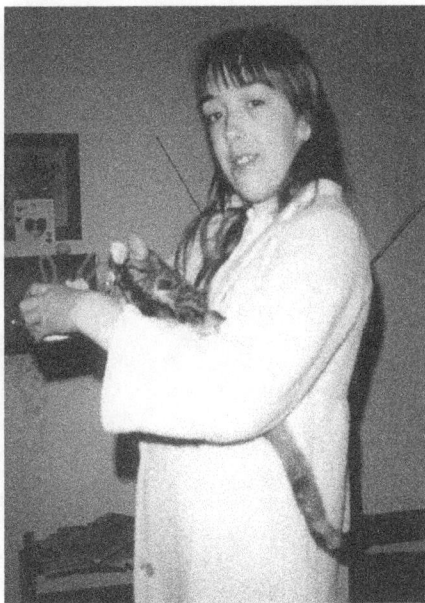

Jen and Rosie

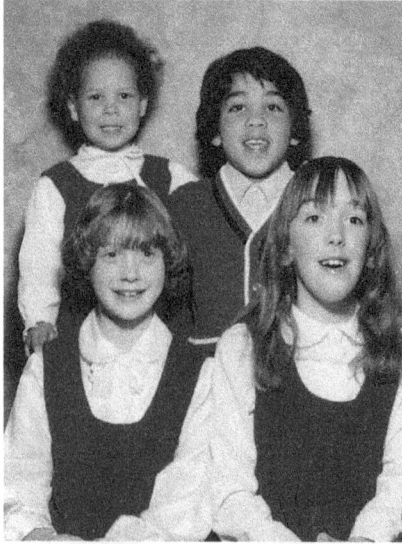

All of our children.

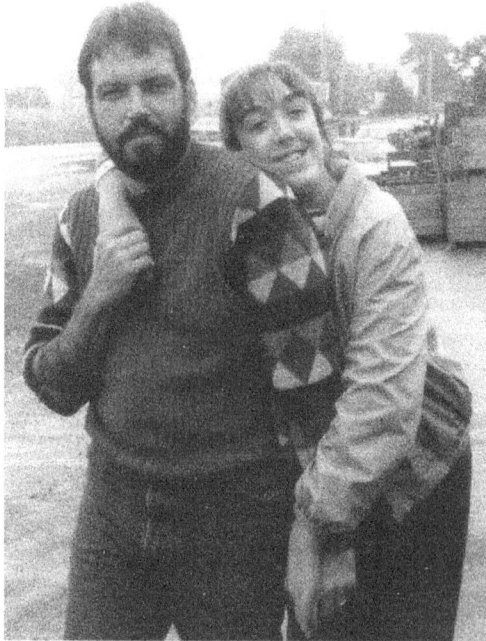

Jen and Dad

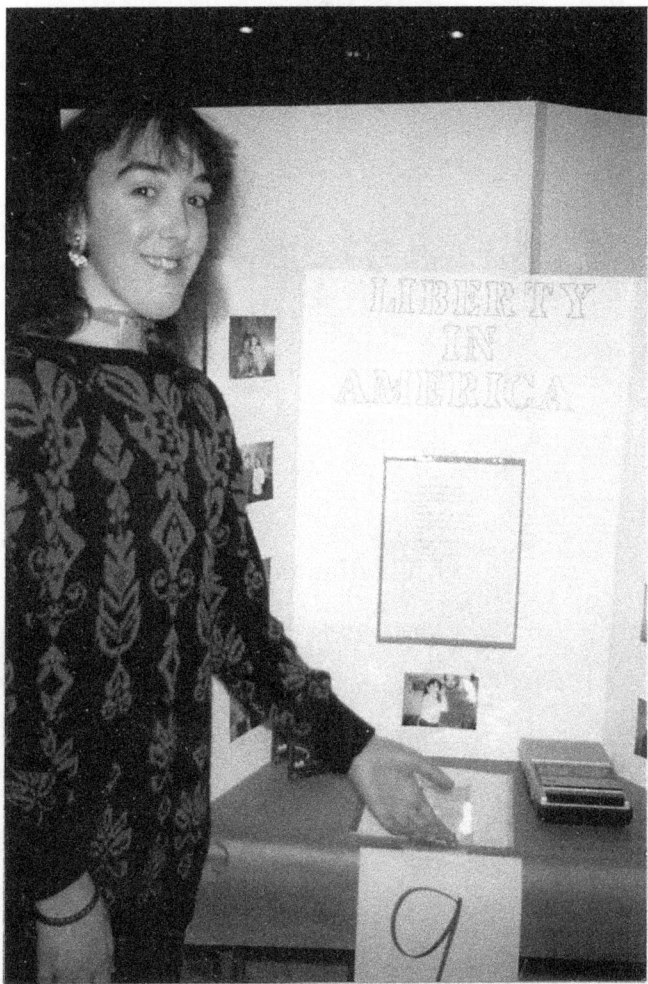

Jen wearing her brace at her eighth grade Science Fair.

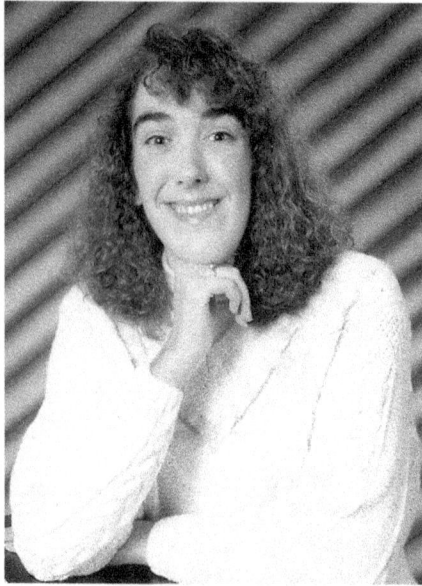

Graduation portrait

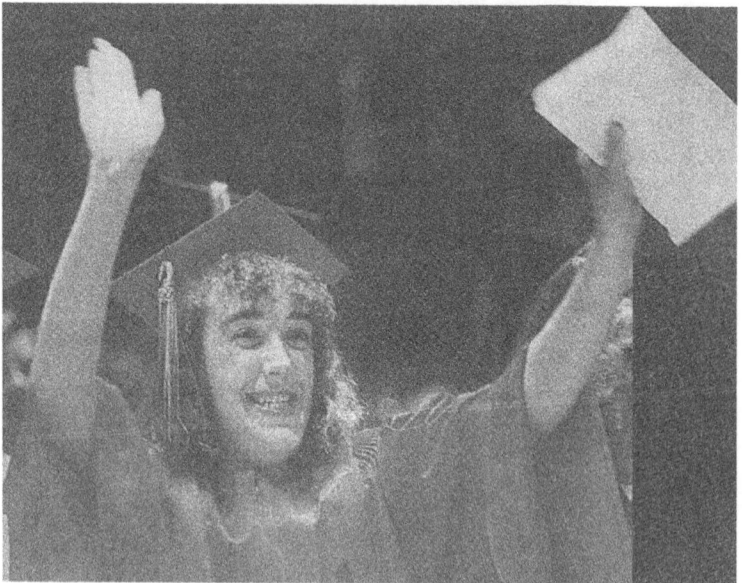

Jen's Commencement celebration made the newspaper.

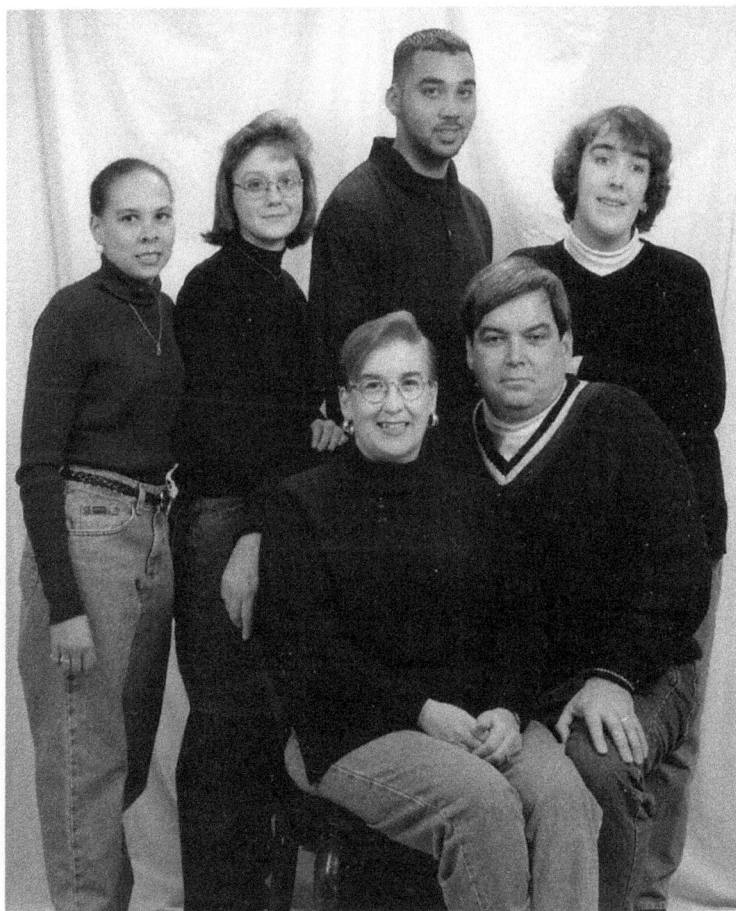

Family portrait, 1997.

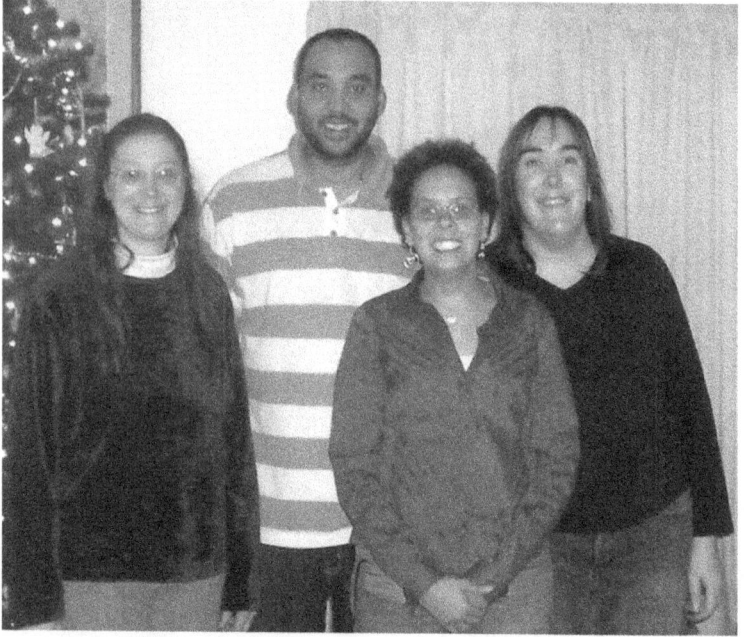

All grown up and home for Christmas.

The Middle Years

If you have four children, you are busy. If you have four children and one has disabilities, you are busier. So the years passed quickly, filled with all the joy and pain that children bring you. Filled with a thousand tasks, a thousand worries, and a thousand hugs. It was mostly a sweet time. A good time. For every hurtful day there was a day full of happiness. We watched all the children grow and enjoyed seeing who they were becoming. Sometimes they stumbled but they always got up and went on. Jennica was no exception.

Most of Jennie's teachers were kind and hard working. Eager to help her and to do a little extra to make school a good place for her. Occasionally though, she would have a teacher that was uncomfortable with who Jennica was. Uncomfortable working with a child with the challenges she had. Those would be years full of stress and meetings. Years where we sat and listened to teachers telling us things we already knew. Things we lived with but things they had only recently discovered. I guess they felt they could help us by bringing these problems to our attention. Mostly we sat, nodded, and sympathized. They were able to express all of their concerns and then life would go on. Some years it was more difficult. Years when we worried that the teacher was working to have Jennica removed from their class, from the school. We knew her rights and we came prepared with information, tape recorders, and resolve. Somehow we made our way through those years, just adding some fresh hurts, some new disappointments in people, but moving forward as always. Most of the stress would fall on us, her parents, and we tried to shield Jennica from it. She remained a happy child. A child who believed that she could do anything. We knew her limitations, both physical and mental, but we also knew her spirit and we cheered her on.

In addition to school, Jennica received two types of therapy for many years. There was speech therapy, both at school and at a private location, and there was occupational therapy, at a children's center. We found a wonderful woman who believed in a type of O.T. called Sensory Integration. At first she was Jennica's therapist at the center and then later she treated Jennie in our home. We purchased or built the equipment she needed and set it up in the family room. There were scooter boards, nets hanging from the ceiling, large therapy balls, and rocker platforms. Not everyone's home is so decorated, but ours was. The therapist was encouraging with Jennie and with us, always trying new methods, working on Jennica's balance and strength. On her manual dexterity. She even worked on more subtle problems like Jennie's hypersensitivity to touch and Jennica's anxiety about schedules. She would make charts about future events and discuss ways Jennie could deal with anxiety. She was a jewel. If you have a disabled child you meet people that can hurt you immeasurably and people that uplift you. This woman lifted the whole family up, in more ways than it is possible to discuss. Her cheerful spirit offered healing to a family that needed it. She worked with Jennie until Jen was thirteen and she felt there would be no further benefit, but she remained in our lives for many years to come and Jennie loved her dearly. She did one more thing. She repeatedly told me that I should write a book about Jennica. Though I couldn't follow her advice then, I remembered it.

At thirteen Jennica was in middle school. She had encountered some obstacles there, such as working the combination lock on her locker. The administration was firm that she must be able to use this lock and so she struggled and we practiced and she struggled some more. The school said it would not be fair to allow anything else. We wondered what was fair about her condition and thought that fair would be giving her what she needed. Then one day an angel in the form of a custodian told me he could remove the combination lock and replace it with a padlock. One that used a key. Once again the administration bulked but it was within her legal rights and that is how she managed lockers from that point on. There were also the stairs at the school. Three floors of them and Jennica, in spite of her balance and muscle problems, did well on them most of the time. One day though, in the middle of a crowd of energetic and impatient students, she lost her footing and fell down a flight of these stairs. We had worried about this happening but were told she must be able to use them. No exceptions could be made. Fortunately she was not seriously hurt and the school then decided to allow her to leave class a minute before the other students to avoid this happening again. And it didn't.

Something did happen when she was thirteen that tested our strength and hers. She had been diagnosed with scoliosis years before and the doctors had been watching her back carefully as she grew. She had an S shaped curve and they told us if it became severe she would have to have it treated. Scoliosis runs in both of our families and with her low muscle tone it was much more problematic. Every few months she was examined by a specialist and x-rayed. I grew concerned about the amount of radiation Jennica had been exposed to in her short life, with many scans, many x-rays for various problems, and now frequent ones for her back. I stopped having her x-rayed for standard dental appointments and questioned every one her doctors ordered. Someone had to look at the big picture of Jennica's health and it seemed that I was that person. On one fateful day those dreaded x-ray's revealed her two curves had reached a severity that had to be treated.

How do you put a young girl who is just starting to mature, and is already so keenly aware of her differences, in a brace that runs from just under her chin to the bottom of her hips? Four metal bars running the length of the brace. The top forced her head up and fit snugly under her chin and the bottom was a stiff leather corset that had been created by a craftsman just for her. She wore that instrument of torture twenty three hours of each day, taking it off only for bathing. Because of the bulky nature of this brace she had to have bigger and stretchy clothing, and still it was a problem with the screws often ripping her blouses. So our daughter spent her early teens even more uncomfortable. Even more aware of her differences. For the most part she did it with strength and grace. She never said she wouldn't wear it but she did say she hated it. She did say how hot and uncomfortable it was. She wore the brace each day. All day. For almost two years. And we prayed it would stop the curvature.

Jennica graduated from the eighth grade in that brace. She was thrilled to be graduating and we were happy to see this day arrive for her. She loved celebrations of all kinds. Days that were special and brought a little extra happiness to her life. She needed celebrations because life was often a struggle, but if there was a reason to celebrate, she was there. Usually at the head of the line for the cake! And always with a lovely smile. Her graduation was no exception. We found a pretty peach colored dress that would accommodate the brace, I did her long hair in soft curls, we added a touch of lip-gloss, and she was ready. Part of her excitement was probably for the attention and for the cake, but most of it was because there was a special eighth grade dance following the ceremony. Brace or not, Jennie loved to dance. She loved the music. So she walked across the stage in her brace, she danced in her brace, and she complained not one time. We, her family, watched her that night with a mixture of emotions but mostly with pride.

Soon after her graduation we were told that the brace was not working and her curvature was so severe it was a danger to her health. Looking at the x-rays I saw the curve that was threatening her life. Her spine not only curved into the S, it was rotating. Spirally around, threatening her internal organs. It had to be corrected with surgery and so we were sent to a specialist at a nearby world renowned hospital. The physician was personable and kind. He was also firm as he explained what must be done. As he explained the surgery, we listened with fear. If we had known exactly how horrible the surgery was, we might have been overcome by that fear. As it was, we scheduled the operation for that summer when I was off from teaching and when I could have the other children taken care of by relatives without missing their school.

Jennica was allowed to discard the brace. She had worn it for all of that time, suffering in so many ways, and it had failed her. She hated it. We hated it. We talked of having a burning party but simply disposed of the heavy, ugly, failure. It was difficult to be happy about its absence knowing what lie ahead but she made the most of the days she had before entering the hospital. She swam and rode her bicycle. She enjoyed the luxurious freedom of sleeping without metal bars poking into her. We all tried to make these days happy, knowing the surgery was next.

The day came, no matter how hard we had tried to wish it away. The surgery took over six hours. The surgeon took bone from her hip and used it to fuse her spine. Top to bottom. Each vertebrae was scraped and a chip of the hip bone inserted so that it would grow and fuse her spine into one long piece of bone. Lining both sides of her spine were Harrington rods, metal rods that were several inches long. These were fastened into her spine with metal hooks. She lie on her stomach in the operating room with her spine straightened out and the hardware going in. Such long hours went by as we prayed, waited, and hoped that all would be well. I don't remember much conversation between John and I. We were beyond that. We simply waited quietly, grateful for the occasional updates given to us by an assistant.

At last the doctor came out and told us the

operation had gone well and that Jennica was in the recovery room. He warned us that she was on a respirator and would remain on it for some time. He warned us that she would be in severe pain when the anesthesia wore off. He told us that they had given her three units of blood during the surgery because of bleeding. This was blood that Jennica had donated prior to the surgery, at great expense because of poor veins and painful prodding. Let me say that being warned is not really so helpful.

When we were allowed into the recovery room she was just waking a little. She was heavily sedated but not so heavily that she wasn't able to point to the tube running into her lungs and motion she wanted it out. Now. I remember being so relieved that she had made it through the surgery and though we hated to see her like this, she was here. And she was strong enough to want that tube out. Over and over she asked by gestures, by facial expressions. Then we were asked to leave so they could attend to her. I don't know what was worse. Leaving her or watching her struggle.

The following day she did get off of the respirator and was moved into a room. While this was a relief, we remained concerned about many things. One was her heart. It was racing and irregular. She was in such severe pain that to say our hearts were broken would be the biggest of understatements. Her condition did not improve as expected and the medical staff did not know what was causing the problems with her heart. Jennica could talk now. Through the pain medicine. Through a scratchy throat, came crying and words that broke my heart then and remain written on it still. She asked us how we could have allowed this surgery if we really loved her. She knew something was very wrong and kept repeating that she, at fifteen, was too young to die. No child should have to go through that and no parent should have to hear words like that. You simply can't be the same person afterwards.

Finally the doctors realized that her heart was in distress because she needed another transfusion. There was no more blood banked and so my husband, who was the same type, donated one unit. The other two were donated blood from strangers. We were worried and afraid because at that time Aids and other blood borne diseases could not be tested for with great accuracy, but there was no choice. They gave her the three additional units of blood and her heart was restored to it's normal functioning. Of course we were relieved but we were also angry. Why hadn't they tested her blood gases sooner after the surgery? Why did it take days of additional suffering for someone to simply do their job. These were questions we asked ourselves but only briefly and then we returned to caring for her as she struggled with her intense pain. John had to return home to make sure all was well with the other children and he had to return to work. So I stayed. I slept in a chair by her bed each night for the two weeks she was a patient. I watched over her and tried to comfort her. Tried to assure her that she would feel better soon. She was simply too frightened and in too much pain for me to leave her for more than a quick shower. That was the summer of 1988. It was one of the hottest summers on record, with days often in the hundreds. There was also a drought, making the earth turn brown and lifeless. Inside the hospital I placed my hands on the windows and felt the   intense heat of that summer and thought it matched the hell inside Jennie's room.

Her sister, Jonna remembers, visiting Jennica there. My parents, who were helping watch the children, brought the children to the hospital to see Jennie. Jonna, the youngest at ten, remembers how hard that visit was. She was happy to see her sister, and to know where she was, but when she walked into Jennie's room she saw the pink stuffed animal that Jennica had taken with her to the hospital. She saw it and she saw the blood on it. Seeing her sister in pain and the blood on the animal was a lot to take in when you are a little girl. I think, I hope, we were right to have the children visit, but when she shared her memories as an adult, it made me sad for her and for everyone else in the family. I know Jennie's grandparents were distraught over seeing their first grandchild lying there looking so very ill. I know her uncles and aunts felt the same. I'm quite sure it was a sight that no one really wanted to see, but there it was, and when they left, there we were. Jennica and I.

Jennica spent two weeks in that room. The pain remained a monster that had taken over her body. She couldn't eat. She slept only briefly and when her pain medication was at its peak. The girl who always smiled and was cheerful, had become a person deeply depressed and withdrawn. As difficult as it was to watch her pain, it was also hard to see her so sad. Her words about how we could "do this to her if we loved her", continually rang in my ears and I questioned what we had allowed. Was it the only way? Was it worth what she was enduring? There was no going back though and I could only pray for her and be there for her.

She was healing, and despite her discomfort things were progressing, and so they sent her home. During her last days at the hospital the pain was managed by the narcotics they gave her and she remained on those at home. She was so fragile and ill that she needed someone with her at all times and for a time I could do that. We brought her home and got her settled in her room. We brought the other children home from their cousins and grandparents and we tried to return to our normal life. Coming home was good for her spirits and though she still wouldn't eat, I felt that she was improving each day. When the time came for me to return to teaching I hired the college age daughter of a colleague to be with Jennica during the day. My colleague was the gentlest and kindest of men and his daughter proved to be the same. In addition, Jennie felt like she had a friend with her and during that month, things improved. Her spirits improved and with that her appetite. She was still thin, but now there was sometimes a smile on her face, usually because of her caregiver. Sometimes because of her siblings. She walked a little around the house and sometimes even into the yard. She walked with stiff, tender steps. Because of her back being fused from her neck to her hips, her walk was awkward, but she was walking and beginning to believe that life was going to get better for her. Day by day she improved that autumn, my favorite season, with the leaves turning vivid shades of red and gold and the air growing crisp. Jennica returned to us that fall. Never to be exactly the same, but she returned, giving me one more reason to love the season.

High School, Growing up, and New Challenges

Eventually Jennie also returned to school. High School. She was thrilled that she was a freshman and we were delighted that she was feeling well enough to attend. She began with half days and before long she was a full time student. Jennica was in a resource room for English and Math but all of her other classes were the regular curriculum. As always, she was a dedicated student. She read and underlined. She took notes on the computer. She listened in class. And she did well. Each grading period she was on the honor or merit roll. It seemed that all the hard work she had done for all those previous years was paying off in high school. She enjoyed her classes and many extra-curricular activities. She was on student council. She sang in the choir, she joined the AFS club, and was even the manager of the softball team. The sunny smile was back and she had a friendly relationship with all of the students. It didn't matter who they were, Jennica liked them and most of her classmates liked her back.

It was Jennica's cheerful nature that made school a positive experience for her but sometimes that wasn't enough. Most teachers liked her, even calling us to tell us how much they appreciated her effort. How much they enjoyed her in class and admired her spirit. That was the norm but there were exceptions. For example there was a history teacher who told my husband that Jennie disgusted him. That it was difficult for him to look at her. I'm not sure how John walked out of that conference without severely injuring this man but I suspect he restrained only because he didn't want to make life even more difficult for Jennie. He never forgot that night and he spoke to the administration about the issue. I guess we could keep it in perspective because of the many other teachers who were sensitive and supporting but the cruelty that some people are capable of never stopped surprising us.

Jennica's social life at school was complicated. She had positive relationships with most of the students but that didn't mean she was invited to parties or out on dates. She had classmates who would sit with her at lunch or sometimes invite her to their homes or to a special event. She did not have a normal high school experience and I suspect that there were times that she was lonely but most often she was content. It helped that her brother joined her at the high school when she was a sophomore. No one could make Jennica laugh like Joshua could and each day she began school with a smile because of him.

I was working at the middle school during this time and each morning I dropped Jennica and Joshua off at the high school on my way to work. Joshua would begin teasing her as they left my van, telling her she was stinky. Then he often gave her a kiss and sent her on her way. Sometimes I saw him bend down to retie her shoelaces that refused to stay tied. I watched their eyes meet as he stood up. I saw the smiles they shared and I was as proud of him as he was proud of her.

High school was a time of pride and it was still flavored with a little hope for a happy life for Jennica. Watching her study, seeing the care she put into her appearance, listening to the dreams she still dreamed, it was easy to be hopeful. Our goals and plans for Jennica had slowly changed since her birth. Gone was the belief that she could have it all. Slowly we let go until by high school we hoped just for a modified life. Still independent, still a fulfilling job, still hope for life with a loving partner. As long as she smiled, it was enough for us. It was different, but it was enough.

Still there were days where neither Jennie or I smiled. These were days when there was no denying that she had been cheated of a "normal" life. It seemed that formal dances were the most difficult for her. She wanted a pretty dress and flowers. She wanted a boyfriend and all that went with that. She watched classmates living her dream and it hurt. It hurt her and it hurt me. Parents dream for their children. It's natural. We think of their lives and wonder what they will do. What they will be interested in. What they will excel at. My dreams for Jennie were more simple. I dreamed that she would have some opportunities and some happiness. When situations occurred in her life where her losses were apparent, we mourned. All of us. And the older she became the more difficult it was to make things better or even distract her. These were times of great sadness and frustration. Times of sleepless nights for me and a mixture of angst and anxiety for Jennica. Once, with hard work and imagination, we were able to make her dream come true by inviting a young man, who was also disabled, to her Junior prom. She had met him at her summer camp and they wrote and kept in touch. We contacted his parents and explained the situation to them. They were delighted to help her and also give their son a chance to attend this special occasion. A chance to experience something most young people do. And so we went shopping and threw the budget to the wind when we found a beautiful soft pink satin dress with beading and sparkles. Jennica beamed as she spun around in it. Her head full of fluffy dreams and her heart full of expectations.

The night arrived, along with her friend. I dare say he was a bit frightened by his overeager date but still he looked pleased to be there. He came armed with a corsage and a shy smile for Jennica who was eager to leave and to show him off. She looked pretty in her finery and her excitement, and so, off they went. Driven by myself. I didn't stay, so I can not say for certain, but it appeared that they had a good time. I believe that in her mind it was a success. When I returned to pick them up Jennie's date still seemed a bit uncertain as to what had happened, and how he had gotten into this situation, but Jennica clutched his arm and escorted him out to the car. There they were. Slightly worse for wear. A little disheveled; him standing several inches shorter than Jennica, she standing in her stocking feet, most unhappy with her dancing shoes, but they stood there. Triumphant. She had gone to her prom. As always, Jennie's version was a little different. A little sadder. But she had made it happen and she was content.

Jennica had a desire to be happy. Obstacles that might have stopped other people simply slowed her down. Her father often told me that if he had her problems he would be found in a corner. Sucking his thumb. I laughed at him but I understood. Jennica was strong. She believed in herself. She believed in her capabilities. It wasn't that she was unaware of her differences; she often discussed prejudice with us. When she encountered it, she recognized it. But she also recognized it as their problem. Not hers. She loved life and choose not to focus on the few people who were unkind, negative, or even cruel. She had an appetite for living that amazed us. I should have known she was like that when she first requested dance classes and refused to believe she shouldn't have them. She made that happen and she was determined to make her other dreams come true too. We tried not to stand in her way, encouraging her when she struggled, comforting her when she was hurt, and cheering her on when she was triumphant.

Jennica was good at cheering people on too. She loved to cheer on her brother and sisters. I often wondered how she felt when she saw them doing things so easily. Physically, socially, educationally. Of course they had problems too but they paled in comparison to hers. I watched her face, looking for jealousy when her siblings received invitations for overnights or parties. When they played in orchestras or were active in sports. When the phone rang for them and not for her. I watched but I never saw it. Instead I saw happiness for them on her face. I have to believe there was some sadness in her heart. Some hurt. But I don't believe there was jealousy. She loved them. She more than loved them, she adored them, and when something good happened to them, she rejoiced. I may have struggled more than she did. I was conflicted. I was delighted for every good thing my other children experienced but I couldn't help wishing Jennie could have the same. I couldn't help wishing life wasn't so very difficult for her no matter how hard she worked at everything.

        I seldom saw Jennie angry. It just wasn't her nature but occasionally it happened and when it did she was usually justified. It was when she recognized discrimination that I saw the fire in her eyes. It happened. It was a fact of life. There were many small things but sometimes there were important things that happened that showed how insensitive some people were capable of being. When Jennica was in high school she received a letter saying that she was being considered for the National Honor Society. The letter listed the requirements, and though I was initially surprised, I realized that she met all of the items listed. She was in the top ten percent of her class. She was active in school functions. She did community work, working in a local nursing home every week during a social hour. I assumed that the school was well aware of her differences but must also be aware of her eligibility. Jennie was so proud, it seemed that all of her academic diligence was paying off. That it was going to be recognized as it was in students without disabilities. Weeks went by and then one sad day she received another letter telling her she was not accepted. She was furious, calling it what it was, discrimination. Of course she was right. There was nothing we could say or do to make this right for her. Along with my own disappointment and anger, I couldn't help but wonder why they ever sent the first letter. Why set her up for such hurt? The committee's answer was that she took easier courses. Period. She had taken some core subjects in a resource room for students with Learning Disabilities but most of her work was done in regular classes and it was the same curriculum that all students took for graduation. She had over a 3.2 grade point average. It simply boiled down to her condition. She knew it, we knew it, and probably some of the school staff knew it, but the person who was in charge denied it. That rejection might have been the first break in her confidence. The first crack in her positive outlook and her belief that she was going to be accepted in the world. It demonstrated beyond a doubt that giving her all was not going to be good enough.

Jennie didn't bounce back quickly from that experience. It was a deep wound and an unnecessary one, but senior year was upon her and there were many new things to focus on and to be excited about. There were senior pictures. There were graduation activities being planned. There was the heady pleasure of being a senior. Jennica enjoyed her year. I know she felt proud of coming this far. Through both health and learning problems. She had made it.

As the year progressed she listened to her classmates discuss college and she was determined she could go to college too. We knew it wasn't that simple but we began looking for a college or program that would accept Jennica and we soon discovered it wasn't an easy task.

The local junior college seemed to the most obvious choice. They had a program for students who had learning disabilities which included tutors and classroom accommodations. What we discovered was they were less than eager to work with a student who had multiple problems. After frustrating meetings and feeling unwelcome, we decided perhaps there was something better out there. A better fit.

We discovered a "college" in a large city that claimed to have a program for learning disabled students. It was a short program but they claimed it would educate them for a career. It was connected to another traditional college and said it offered the disabled students a similar experience . We were hopeful and cautiously excited. We decided to fly there to see what the program was really like. We made a little vacation of it and flew the whole family into the city and off to an upscale hotel. The children had grown up in a small town so visiting this area was exciting for all of them. Of course the most excited was Jennica. Me? Well, I crossed my fingers and hoped.

The school was in a lovely area of the city and it did have a connection to a well known college. Then we entered the classrooms. I was tying to be open minded but I was surprised. The population of students appeared to be much lower functioning intellectually than Jennie. The class was not a traditional class but more of a hands on setting. Neither of these things were necessarily a problem. But. The training was for manual jobs that, in my mind, required more physical strength than Jennie had. In addition, students received a small amount of in-class training and then were sent out on the city buses to various locations for on-the-job experience. When the training ended they would receive help to find jobs in that city. I couldn't see this working. At all. It appeared to me that this was a program offered to parents who wanted to pretend their children went away to school like other people's children but in actuality were participating in a vocational program with severe limitations. What would

Jennica have that would help her when she was done? She wasn't able to live independently in that city so far away. The actual training was minimal and not really suitable for her. I couldn't see this as an option.

So, sometimes we make decisions that we aren't totally sure about simply because decisions have to be made. Jennica wanted to go to "college" like her school friends. She, as always, longed for a normal life and if this was as close as she could get, she would take it. John was unsure. I know he wanted to please Jennie. To give her what she wanted. I don't believe he was impressed by the program and had many unanswered questions himself. I remember that her brother had immediately ruled the program out after seeing the current students. He couldn't see Jennica fitting in with these young people who seemed to be so much lower functioning than his sister. I had little doubt this wasn't the situation for my daughter but that didn't make it any easier to tell her that. Not a bit easier.

Jennica had learned to fight for what she wanted. Time after time. And so she fought for attending this school. If my only job as her mother was to please her, to satisfy this immediate desire, then I should have said yes. Right or wrong, I didn't. I could find no acceptable alternative but I couldn't convince myself that just because this school would accept her, it was right for her. So for the first time in her life, I did not support her. I did not work to make something happen for her. Sometimes I question myself now but I honestly think I would make the same decision if the situation presented itself again. The search now began for an alternative.

Her school suggested the Bureau of Vocational

Rehabilitation (BVR). It was a support and placement group that helped out people with some type of disability. We were told they provided both training and placement for people like Jennica. Hoping that this would be an opportunity for her we enrolled her for the following year and she continued on with her senior year.

In many ways it was a good year but in some ways it was a peek into the future. Jennica was still determined to have the life she wanted but she was starting to understand that there would be obstacles in her way. There had been the problems with the Honor Society. There was the struggle to find some type of secondary education. There remained the heartbreak of a limited social life and that elusive boyfriend and yet there were happy and proud days her senior year.

Jennica did not have a date for her senior prom. It frustrated and saddened her until her brother and his girlfriend came to her rescue. They decided that she would attend the prom with them. Loving both her brother and his girlfriend, Jennie agreed. On that night the three of them climbed into the car and headed for a night of dancing and fun. Joshua not only took her, his friends danced with her. Josh and his date danced with her. It might not have been the night she dreamed of, but it was a good night. A happy night. I was proud of her brother and relieved that what could have been another disappointing night for Jennie, wasn't.

As graduation day neared Jennica had another dream and that was to speak at her graduation ceremony. As in most schools, the valedictorian and the class president spoke but in Jennica's school they also picked another student or two and Jennie was determined she would be one of those. She had a staff member at the high school work with her helping prepare her speech. We knew nothing about it, just that she was practicing with the kind man who had offered to help her.

That special night arrived, along with the heat and humidity that always seems to accompany a high school graduation. The ceremony was held in an imposing college chapel and the pews were filled. The balcony was filled. Proud parents, grandparents, siblings, uncles, aunts, and friends, filled this lovely old structure. In the front, spread across the stage were the graduates dressed in their bright red caps and gowns. They all looked excited, proud, and freshly scrubbed; ready for the next chapter in their lives. The organ music played and filled the building as we fanned ourselves and smiled. We clapped for each student, for each administrator, and especially for our daughter. Our daughter who had begun her life with a struggle and whose life remained a struggle. Our daughter who refused to be stopped and who had overcome most of the barriers life had put in her way. She walked proudly to the podium when it was her turn to speak and she spoke clearly and sweetly to the hundreds of people in front of her. She thanked all those who had helped her in her life and made this moment possible for her. She spoke of her happiness at graduating. She ended by thanking us, her parents, for being there for her. She stood tall and again thanked the audience. There was a brief silence and then applause. Thunderous applause. The gentle man who had helped her prepare her speech stood up and the rest of the audience followed. I don't know what everyone else felt that night, though I do believe they were moved, but I know that the tears I shed were happy tears. Proud tears. I knew it was the end of that chapter in her life and she had ended it with pride. The next day's paper featured a picture of Jennica on the stage with a huge smile. Nothing could have pleased her more.

Life After School

As every parent knows, watching your child leave school and become an adult is not easy. You watch them and you worry. You long for the days when you could dry their tears and make things better. And yet, with most children you have a sense of pride as you watch them become independent and strong. You know it's time they leave the nest and begin the great adventure of their own life. With Jennica it was different. We watched as she tried to become a part of the world beyond school. We watched as she was rejected by a society that had no tolerance for differences. No appreciation for a person, like Jennica, who just wanted to have a life too.

In Jennica's senior year she had arranged to work with the local BVR. They had promised her job training followed by job placement using her new skills. While Jennie had dreamed of college, this program offered her hope and a chance of learning a skill and so she was eager to begin.

After meetings with their personnel, and some evaluations, she was enrolled in a program that trained her to work in a deli and in a small health food grocery. It was in the city and so she was transported there each day where she was taught to work filling deli orders, restocking shelves, and working with customers. It was a friendly environment and Jennie thrived there. She enjoyed working with the staff and they enjoyed her. She was happy and therefore we were happy too. Her training was a nine month process and during that time life was hopeful and smooth. At the end of her training Jennica received a document which stated she had successfully completed the program. Adding to her feeling of pride were the encouraging words of the program director who told us that she had completed the program more skillfully than any of her predecessors. She was now ready for the next step in her life. Employment.

We were certainly optimistic about her finding work with the recommendation of her trainers. Overly optimistic it soon became apparent. The staff member from the BVR that was assigned to find Jennie appropriate work was a cold person who never seemed to really show any interest or feelings about Jennica or her job hunt. Her efforts produced this: a job at a local restaurant washing dishes for about three hours per week. If she was needed. We were all disappointed and saddened that a program that had started out so promising, ended like this. Case closed. She was employed.

While the case might have been closed for the agency, Jennica's life was still wide open and she needed work. She needed a purpose, a reason to get up each morning and to feel like a productive citizen. We were out of ideas and feeling despair as we watched our once cheerful daughter's frustration. That's when two friends stepped in. People who knew Jennica and decided to support her in her job quest. There was a grocery store in our town that we had thought perfect for Jen and her training. Again and again Jennica applied there. Each time she was told they were not hiring and yet we saw new people begin working there. That's when Jennica's supporters stepped in. They recognized discrimination when they saw it and they saw it. They approached the owner of the store and informed him that if Jennica was not hired for the next opening they would be contacting officials that protected the rights of the disabled. She was hired the next day.

It was perfect. This was something Jen knew. Something she was trained for. She would be able to show them she was capable and so she began. No one was ever more excited about the prospect of wearing a produce apron then Jennica. And then reality reared it's ugly head. The store had no intention of really letting Jennica work there. They might be forced to follow the letter of the law, but they could ignore the spirit of it. I remember the heavy feeling that covered me when I realized that they were not going to let Jennica stay there. They refused to let her do anything. She stood there. We contacted the BVR, and they reluctantly reopened her case so that a job coach could be provided for Jennie. This job coach was to insure that Jen's work would be satisfactory. That there would be no risk to the grocery. And still she was not given a chance. One day Jennica's coach shared with us what had been said to her. That they considered the coach a glorified babysitter for Jennie and that they were not going to allow Jen to stay beyond the probationary period. That had been their plan from the first. There would be no produce apron in her future. Such a little dream in a world full of dreams and yet it too was impossible. As I said before, having a child with a challenge will bring the best and the worst of people into your lives. This incident did both. It angered people who knew Jen. Enough that they wanted to fight for her rights. It also introduced us to several kind people at the grocery who were good to Jennica. Unfortunately it brought out the worst in the owners and management. People that refused to see Jennie as a person with capabilities and only saw her as a problem. I felt rather numb about the whole situation. Oh, I was angry. I was angry at the mean spirited people who were blinded by any differences. I was angry at the life Jennica had been given. I was angry, but I was beginning to realize the futility of my anger. Of my efforts. Of Jennica's efforts. Being angry is no way to live a life but I assure you that being numb isn't either, and yet I was both.

Jennie was changing. A change that had begun in high school when she had been rejected by National Honor Society and now continued through each new road block. Through each new situation that revealed the prejudice that was demonstrated against her. She was angry. She spoke of discrimination with fire in her eyes. She knew exactly what was happening to her and though she had never anticipated it, she recognized it and knowing it was directed at her, she began to change. I think of all the things that broke my heart during this time, that was the worst.

John and I were both puzzled as to the next step and for a while we thought about it and tried to make a new plan for what appeared to be a new and very challenging part of Jennie's life. Then one day John came home from work smiling and with good news. He had spoken to his company's cafeteria manager about our daughter and it seemed that she could begin work there. She would not have a glamorous job, it would be scrubbing pots and pans in a dark corner of the kitchen, but it was a beginning. There were promises for advancement. For her to work preparing the salad bar and to be out in the dining room. So, with that in mind, along with the promise of a paycheck, they became a team. Each day John and Jennie would leave early in the morning, drive into the city, and report to their respective jobs. It started out with so much promise. For all of us.

Though I doubt that Jen ever really enjoyed scrubbing pans, she did her best, she did it cheerfully, and every two weeks she brought home a nice paycheck. Now that she loved. She also loved many of the people there and seeing her father during lunch time. Jennica is a person who dreams. She never wanted to accept limitations and being a dishwasher was certainly not on her dream list but she was learning that she was going to have to downsize her dreams. Not an easy transition but she tried.

For almost a year and a half she tried. Every morning she got ready, said goodbye, and left for work with her father. She left in the red car she had convinced her Dad they needed for work. Jennica loves a sporty red car! Each day she left with a little less excitement and with a little more sadness. Her smile disappeared and she withdrew more each day. It was a year and a half of promises for promotions that never materialized. It was a year and a half of growing discontent and frustration for Jennica who saw nothing but a corner of a kitchen and greasy pans. Finally after John confronted her boss about why Jennica had not been moved to the salad bar as promised he was told that they felt that she would make the customers uncomfortable with her appearance. That, basically, she would be unappetizing. Things went downhill quickly after that. Jennica became more depressed, stopped making any effort, and was let go.

John shared what had happened to Jennie with his own boss and once again he was reminded of the good in the world. This man was full of compassion, perhaps because he had almost lost a son to cancer and knew the agony a parent can go through with a hurting child. Perhaps because he was just a good man. Whatever the reason, he offered to invent a job for Jennica. To let her do simple office jobs. Some filing, some copying, some mail delivery. John was so touched that he accepted even though he was not certain Jennica could be successful in her present state of mind. Fresh out of high school, yes, but now, she was not in good shape.

It was a time of struggle. The changes that had begun in the person Jennica was, continued. None were positive. Not only was Jennica dealing with a world that didn't value her, she was dealing with a medication problem that was increasing her depression. It was also causing insomnia, aggravation, and anorexia. This was the result of a change in a seizure drug she had taken for nearly two decades. Her doctor had switched her from a liquid form to a pill that claimed to be the same medicine but without the horrid taste. It soon became apparent that she did not metabolize the pill in the same way as her old medication. Her doctor did not believe the drug change was causing her problems but when I discussed it with her pharmacist he said he had heard of such cases. He got out the literature about this new drug and in it was a list of every symptom Jennica had developed. With this information in hand, I returned to her physician who reluctantly changed her back to the liquid form of the drug. This was a medication that built up in her body over weeks and months and it left that slowly too.

During this time I took her to a psychiatrist who diagnosed her with situational depression. She warned me that if it was not alleviated soon it could become a chronic condition. She proved to be right. That day it was hard to believe that my daughter, the eternal optimist, could lose her sunny smile forever. I'm glad I couldn't see into the future because I still needed a little hope. Just a little.

While Jennica was happy about this new job she was not stable. She could not concentrate on her work. Her mind was on the heartbreak of her life. On the way the world had treated her. On every hurt she had suffered and every dream she now realized would not be fulfilled. It was all too much for her. She was up multiple times in the night, often coming into my room to spout out angry words about some new or old pain. She couldn't eat. She became painfully thin and it hurt me to see her fresh sweet face become boney and angular, her legs now no bigger around than her arms. It also surprised me. It surprised me to see the person Jennie had become. My daughter had become a person full of rage. Nothing pleased her. Nothing made her happy. Nothing I did made the huge pain she felt any better.

She had to leave work. We all knew that no matter how touched we were by the man who had tried to help, she just couldn't function there anymore. And so her days began at home.

With the medicine changed she began eating better and even sleeping a bit more peacefully but still the depression continued and the anger just poured out of her. She paced through the house fighting with everyone there. She talked to herself and she withdrew deeper into the pain inside her head. It was difficult to leave her alone and while at work I worried about what she was doing. The only thing I was certain about was the fact I had no answers. Not inside me. Not from the medical community. Not from her regular doctor or her psychiatrist. She fell apart and I watched, trying not to fall apart myself. We were alone then. I have no doubt that people felt badly about Jen. About us. And yet we faced this by ourselves with few offers of relief. Few offers of help for Jennica or us. I knew it was our problem. Our situation, but so often in the isolation of pain I wished for a helping hand from anyone.

I can not imagine the agony that Jennica was going through then. I could see the way it manifested itself but I don't think that anyone could really know what she was feeling. I do know that she must have felt like the world had turned against her. Had ignored her. One day she looked at me in anger and screamed, asking what she was. Was she a shadow person that no one could see? I stopped breathing for just a moment when I heard her words. Partly because of her tortured soul. Partly because I had no answer for her.

The following months brought more outbursts and more withdrawal. Jennie started living inside her own mind. She made up a life that she wanted and she convinced herself it was real. Boyfriends. Careers.

Marriages. She wrote letters to people that made no sense if you didn't understand that she was reinventing her reality. She was rushing to the inevitable and that was hospitalization.

Jennica had fallen apart and we were all falling apart with her. Months of sleepless nights and constant crisis had taken their toll on all of us. John was frustrated, wanting to solve this problem, and he often lost his temper. I couldn't think clearly and had trouble concentrating. Jennica's psychiatrist had no answers and so he suggested we hospitalize her. Truly I can't remember how we felt about the idea of driving our daughter to a mental health facility, but we did it. We were out of energy, hope, and help. So we did it. We took her there, filled out forms, talked to the intake people about the situation and we left her there. I think she was ready. She didn't struggle. Somewhere in her she knew she was out of control and maybe she was relieved at the chance to feel better.

It was a silent drive home. What could be said? We had just committed our daughter. We had admitted defeat. We were numb, exhausted, and feeling nothing much except despair. I slept that night. You might ask how but I had not slept for months. Worry and middle of the night ravings from Jennica had left me tired in body and soul. Of course Jennica wasn't the only thing going on in my life. Work continued each day where I did my best to meet my students' needs. My other children had their own growing up challenges and needed me too. My marriage was suffering from neglect and I couldn't even remember who I was, it had been so long since I had the time or energy to take care of myself. And so, I slept.

It was a brief peace. Though we traveled to the hospital each day, it was quiet. Nights were undisturbed and we felt Jennica was where she needed to be. It was a fragile peace and one phone call ended it. One frantic phone call from the hospital staff. Jennica was out of control, trying to leave, screaming, crying, and banging on the glass doors of the unit. They wanted us there immediately.

You have probably said something like "it can't get worse than this" sometime in your life. That is certainly how I felt with my daughter in a mental hospital. But I was wrong. It did get worse. When we arrived at the hospital we found Jennica strapped down on a bed with stiff leather cuffs restraining her arms and legs. Staff stood there as she thrashed around yelling and fighting with the restraints. Her eyes were wild with anger and fear, as she looked at me. As she looked at me wanting me to help. I understood how frustrating her behavior had been there, after all I had been living with it for some time. What I didn't understand was why they picked this method of restraining her instead of giving her a drug to calm her. I told them I wanted her to be sedated instead of using the restraints and they agreed. I also talked to Jennica through my own tears, trying to let something positive come from this experience. I told her this was what could happen to her if she couldn't find a different way to handle her anger. That it would be out of my control because they had to stop her. I told her to try to work with the staff and find a better way to deal with her pain. Not to lose control, that I didn't want to see her like this ever again. Then they gave her a drug that allowed her to sleep, they removed the straps and they returned her to her room.

Her psychiatrist resigned. He told us he could not help her. Something that was to be repeated by several more psychiatrists over the years to our frustration. He did refer her to a neurologist that had experience with patients with disabilities. This man brought her a little peace and a little self respect. He treated her with kindness and dignity when he visited her at the hospital and afterwards during her office visits. He also changed her drugs. Removed some, replaced some, and introduced some different ones. In addition he gave us the name of a psychiatrist/neurologist at a nearby famous hospital. He wanted us to take Jennica there and consult with this specialist. It all made sense to us and we relaxed a little with the calming influence of this new doctor. Jennica stayed there for another three weeks while they monitored her reaction to the new drugs. When they discharged her she was not the same person that entered the hospital, nor was she the delightful person she used to be. She was a person in a fog. A calmer person but a person that had neither highs or lows. A person that seldom expressed anger but also seldom smiled. There was no joy in her release. There had been no cure for Jennica, they had simply found a way to control her. And so the ride home that day was as silent as the day we had left her there.

A New Season

Jennica's life had never been an easy one but her spirit, her joy in living, her sense of humor, all made it less of a challenge. For her and for us. She cheered us up with her sunny smile and determination and we cheered her on as she tackled each obstacle in her path. There was a balance of sunny and gray days and there was always the inspiration Jennie provided.

That light was now extinguished. She was withdrawn and depressed. Her dreams were gone and she walked through each day slow with drugs and hopelessness. We watched her; exhausted, sad, and without any idea how to help. Without any idea of how to make this better.

One day, in the middle of this heavy time, the phone rang. It was from a woman who told me she could help with Jennie's situation. She explained that she ran a center for severely disabled adults. It was a place where activities and therapy were provided for people who were not capable of working, or even attending the local workshop for the disabled. Clients were picked up by bus in the morning and returned late in the afternoon. Her idea was that Jennica could attend there while she was in limbo. That she could help the people there and feel like she had a purpose. At that point in time it seemed like an answer to a prayer and the woman I was speaking to was an angel. Jennica was willing to go though she showed little enthusiasm or excitement. She remained both angry and withdrawn. She went, but she went wrapped in sadness and disappointment.

And so this new season began. Jennica went to the haven for people that society had no use for. She went to offer help but, in truth, she was one of those people. During her day she would push wheelchairs, feed clients, sometimes read to someone, or even do a little paperwork. The woman who ran this facility and the staff were kind, compassionate, and selfless. Jennie began to heal. Just a little.

For months Jennica traveled to this center, gaining back a little of her belief in people. A little of her self confidence. Then one day the staff suggested that Jen apply to the local system for disabilities. Most of the clients in this system were mentally retarded but some people, like Jennica, had multiple disabilities. We were told that there had been changes in the law that made Jennica, with her many challenges, eligible for their services. We had mixed feelings about this. Here was our daughter who had graduated in the top ten percent of her high school class, being recommended for a system that was traditionally for people who were much lower functioning than she was. And yet, we were hopeful this would be a place where Jennie could find acceptance. A place where she could relax and not have to be compared to people more fortunate. A place she could find peace.

We began the application process. It involved meetings, testing, and evaluations. We wondered about the I.Q. tests and whether her score would disqualify her, but to our surprise she scored significantly lower than she had in the past. Previously she had tested in the average or low average range but the psychologist explained that her severe depression had, no doubt, lowered this score. With the application completed, we now waited and hoped that this might be a place where Jennica would be welcome.

We all gave a sigh of relief and sent up a prayer of thanks when we were notified of her acceptance. Gone were Jennica's dreams for a normal life. Gone was the belief that with enough effort she could overcome prejudice. What was left was our hope for her peace and a little happiness. That dream remained. It had a new form and a new face but we embraced it and Jennica did the same.

This agency had many facilities. There was a school for younger clients; children who had been identified with significant problems early in their lives. There were workshops that offered a chance for older people to experience work and the pleasure of earning a paycheck. The jobs were piece work and the employees were paid by the amount of work they completed. The work was simple, but real, coming from different industrial companies in the area. The amount of money that could be earned was minuscule but it was important. It served both as incentive and as reward and Jennica was ready to join this workforce. She felt this was a new chance to prove herself. I think she also told herself this was something it wasn't. It is difficult to explain but during this time she still had fantasies running through her head. When questioned about them she could tell you what was real and what wasn't but it seemed she choose to improve on her reality by living in a better place. Her mind.

Each day Jennica went to the workshop. The

building was an attractive, modern structure separated into several different areas. There were conference rooms, offices, therapy rooms, a cafeteria, and the many work stations. The work areas were divided by skill levels and were kept small in size. A dozen or so clients were at each station and with them were two or three workshop employees guiding the clients as they worked. Arranging the current materials necessary for the job. Other supervisors walked the floor making sure both the jobs and the clients were fine. The job stations were in an open, warehouse like environment which added to the feel that this was "real" work. The clients' welfare was important to the staff and they were most often kind and nurturing, which is just what Jennie needed then. She entered this facility with ambition and an eagerness to both do well and to earn money and because of that it was a more peaceful time with her feeling some success.

During this time we used another service provided for clients. We put Jennica's name on their housing list. The agency had many homes where different levels of supervision were supplied to provide a degree of independence for their clients. We had reached the point of acceptance with Jen. We knew she was not going to be able to live a completely independent life and we worried about her future when we were gone. Of course we had always worried about her future, it's what you do when you have a child with challenges, but the experiences we had gone through with her since high school made it even more worrisome. The prospect of us dying and leaving Jennie's care to her siblings was not something we wanted. We didn't want that for Jennica nor her brother and sisters. We hoped that they would all remain close, but because of love, not because of obligation or necessity. Jennica talked about wanting to move out. She had watched both Julie and Joshua leave the nest and she knew that is what grown up children did. Once she, in her typical dramatic fashion, declared that she was the oldest woman alive who still lived with her parents! So it was with her approval that she was put on the waiting list for a new home and we began the wait.

I wish I could say that these changes brought happiness to Jennie. I wish I could say that her big smile and her love of life had returned but that would not be true. The sadness, the restlessness, the anger Jennica had felt the last few years remained. It was just eased a bit. The drugs, the counseling, the stress free workplace helped her function but nothing brought back the daughter we had raised for twenty years. Life had taken her away and I had little hope she would ever return.

This was a lonely time for Jennie. There had always been a little loneliness for her but there were distractions and pleasures for her too. Now there were no social events. No school or neighborhood friends. No schoolwork to occupy her mind. No dreams to focus on. Now there was the workshop and her family and while her family offered love and times of happiness, it also brought her a dose of reality. She watched each sibling going out in the world. She watched them, succeeding and sometimes failing, as they became adults but she knew they were having a normal life. One with new experiences and challenges. She watched them marry and have children. That might have been the most difficult for her to see. She had dreams of a family of her own and it was a difficult dream to give up. I watched her, helpless to make it better. When she was a child I could cheer her up with a party or a new lesson. I could hug her and sing to her and bring her smile back but those days were gone and I was powerless to give her what she wanted. It wasn't mine to give.

Discontent began building in Jennica again as she lost interest in the workshop she attended. Part of the problem was that there was now less work for the clients to do and too many days there was none. The same economy that was causing suffering in the general population was hurting the already hurt people who attended the workshop. Jennica hated going there and finding there was no work, leaving her bored and frustrated all day. She never knew when this would be and so she began refusing to attend. More and more often we could not convince her to go though we stressed that at least she was around other people during the day, even when there wasn't work. Full of new disappointment and continuing depression she again became agitated and often sleepless. Searching for something to be happy about she focused on finding a more grown up place to live. Not with her parents. I knew that she would be happier living where there were other people and where there was fresh staff showing up every eight hours. I was the staff and I needed some help.

I knew the waiting list for housing was long. Years long. I knew there was nothing I could do about that and yet one desperate day I found myself in the office of the woman who ran this entire agency. I found myself with no pride, crying and explaining the life I was living with Jennica. Broken sleep. Constant stress. Explaining how I was powerless to help her with her desire to move on and that I was exhausted. I'm not proud of the woman I was that day and I doubt that the woman I confronted was impressed, but that is who I was at that moment. A woman saddened and sleepless. A woman with no answers for her daughter. A woman begging a stranger to help. No matter how crazy she thought I was, she was kind, soft spoken, compassionate, and she did not call security! Did she offer help? No. She told me sweetly that the list was long and would remain long. That she was sorry.

Perhaps God heard me that day and intervened. I'm sure he would have wanted to save my daughter from a mother who had nothing left to give. Maybe it was circumstance. All I know for certain is soon after this dramatic display of emotion I received a phone call from the agency telling me that they had an opening for Jennie in a home. They told me that there had been sixteen women ahead of Jennica in line for this placement and all of them had turned it down. Now, that might have to be attributed to divine intervention. I asked the appropriate questions about why they turned this home down. About where the home was. About who else lived there. With positive responses to all my questions we scheduled a visit.

All of us were excited. John, Jennica, and myself. And I was stunned. How could sixteen people turn down a chance to live in this house? It was just beyond me. We were invited to join the residents for supper at their home and off we went. With a little worry and a lot of excitement. Jennica was happy. She kept comparing her move to going off to college, which made me sad but it had become the way she handled her life. One part reality with two parts fantasy. It concerned me but I understood it.

The home was a fifteen minute drive from our house. Pulling into the driveway we were pleased to see it was a large, new, two story. The neighborhood was pleasant and clearly a newer development. Jennica was quiet but happy to see how nice both the neighborhood and the house were. We were welcomed inside by the home's staff and its three current residents. They seemed as excited and eager to please as we were. After a brief tour of their home we joined them for a spaghetti dinner served in the kitchen. The residents were women who were ten to twenty years older than Jen, and recognizing this, they immediately treated her like a younger sister. All were very verbal and pleasant. It was obvious that they liked their home and were proud of it. The house had four bedrooms and three bathrooms. It had a large eat in kitchen with a step down living room and a dining room that was functioning as an office on the other side of the cooking area. It also had a laundry room upstairs and a full basement for storage. It was light and open and both John and I felt relief at the atmosphere our daughter would be living in. Jennica acted a bit shy but she was smiling and I'm certain she was excited by this welcome change in her life.

Within a week Jennie had moved into her large, freshly painted room. Her clothes were in her wall length closet along with personal items to decorate her new quarters. We bought her a new double bed and two dressers which Jennica had happily picked out. With that delivered, she was ready. The day we left her there was a bittersweet one. We knew it was the right thing and that she was happy but still there was sadness. There was another emotion with us that day and it was relief. Not only because of the peace we would have after years of turmoil, but from a fear we had had for years. The one that was ever present and had been for most of Jennica's life. What would happen to her when we died. Driving into the city John saw people living on the streets and he was overcome by fear that this could be his daughter's fate. I felt that her siblings would never let that happen but I knew what a strain it would be for them if they were left in charge of her. And so, the thought that I could die in peace now went through my mind. Over and over. I hoped I would be around for a long time but if I wasn't, Jennica was okay. All arrangements had been made and she would have kind people helping her to live her life. In her own home. I could die in peace.

A New Life

Jennica's move to her own home was the beginning of her adult life. An adult life different from yours and mine, but it was the life she was given. No longer was I able to supervise her each day and guide her in her daily living. She was grown and she was more independent. She was responsible for going to work, for cleaning her room and home, for helping with meals and doing her own laundry. In these ways her life was like most twenty-six year old women. The differences were found in more subtle ways.

Her home had staff. People who made sure the home ran smoothly. They assisted with making meals, with supervising chores, and with looking out for the welfare of the women who lived there. They took care of medications and they stayed during the night to insure the safety of the clients. They were also there to provide transportation. The women did not drive so they were dependent on staff to take them where they wanted or needed to be. To grocery shop, to bank, to see doctors, or to just to do some recreational shopping and a meal out: the staff provided the wheels. They often provided something equally important and that was emotional support. Someone to talk to and to share their day with. They were important people in Jen's life and made her new independent life possible.

Most of the staff were kind and caring. All of them were different of course, with their own strengths and weaknesses, but over all good people. One of

Jennica's favorite staff was a retired nurse who was close to her grandmother's age. She was the weekend employee and the women looked forward to her gentle presence at the end of each week. She never failed to treat them with respect and dignity. Even love. Jennica loved her back and was always more content when she was there. Jen enjoyed most of the staff but this woman was special to her.

Of course there were conflicts in the home. Four women living together have conflicts. Four women with various disabilities have perhaps more conflicts. I doubt if it was much different than anyone with roommates but in this case they had to work things out because no one was likely to be leaving. Jennie became closer to one woman there and they sometimes referred to themselves as sisters. She was about ten years older and a lively person, as talkative as Jennica was quiet. She loved dressing up with sparkly accents and a heavy application of makeup that showed the world what she was about. She often made Jennie laugh and she did the same for John and I. We all enjoyed her bubbly personality and we were glad she was living with Jen.

There were occasional conflicts with staff too. As I have said, most were kind and compassionate people but some might have been better suited for other work. There was an occasional cruel word or lack of respect. A cold tone of voice or perhaps a heavy hand instead of gentle guidance. Over the years I saw those people come and go, often weeding themselves out but not before bringing a little more grief to those who didn't need it. All of these issues fell on the shoulders of the lovely young woman who ran the home. I felt both admiration and occasional sympathy as she worked to make the home a positive place to live. I think she also gave Jennica someone to relate to. Perhaps not really as a friend but something approaching that. She was Jennica's age and a spirited woman like Jen. She is still in charge and I am grateful that she continues to be an advocate for my daughter. Some people have a calling for this type of work and she is certainly one of them.

Jennica no longer lived with us but she certainly stayed in touch. Mostly with phone calls. Receiving twenty calls a day was not unusual. I had been her security blanket for over two decades and a change in location had not stopped that. I wish I could say I answered each and every phone call cheerfully, or even answered each call, but I can't. I talked to her several times a day but many calls were repetitive or something that could wait. Perhaps for months! So I took many calls and tried to balance her sanity with my own. Jennie also came home for weekend visits, sleeping in her old room, eating my cooking. Maybe going shopping with me or going for a haircut. She always came for holidays and birthday celebrations and those remained her favorites. No matter how excited she had been to move out, she was always excited to return. Not too much different than how other young people feel. There is always the familiar comfort of home.

While Jennica was adjusting to her new life, I was settling into my own. I was tired. Plain and simple. Just tired. Parents have such an important job raising children. Such a blessed job. And yet it is a job with time limits. It is but a season. Our lives remain forever entwined but the raising is over, with only the love remaining. That is the natural order of things. I was ready to move on and each day I was grateful that we were able to watch our daughter move on too. Not in the way I had dreamed of. Not in the way she had dreamed of. And yet it was moving on. I like to believe that there is happiness in her future. That all the strength, joy, and love of life, that made her who she was can be rekindled and she will find a way to be happy. That she will find a way to dance.

My Hopes and Wishes

No one's life is complete until they depart this earth. Jennica is no different. Her life remains a work in progress. She struggles and she triumphs. She accepts and she rebels. She is still a young woman and I have hopes that she will find the happiness that has been so elusive for her. That she will find the acceptance she longs for. I have hopes she will rise above those who would pull her down and that she will find a way to be peaceful with who she is. A beautiful and brave woman.